Shoulder Arthroscopy

Olivier Courage

Shoulder Arthroscopy

How to Succeed!

With Forewords by Stephen S. Burkhart
Philippe Hardy

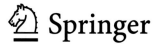 Springer

Olivier Courage
Générale de Santé Hopital privé de
l'Estuaire
Le Havre
France

Translation from the French language edition "Comment réussir ses arthroscopies d'épaules?" by Olivier Courage © Sauramps Medical, Montpellier, 2014; ISBN 9782840239130

Additional material to this book can be downloaded from http://extras.springer.com

ISBN 978-3-319-23647-6   ISBN 978-3-319-23648-3   (eBook)
DOI 10.1007/978-3-319-23648-3

Library of Congress Control Number: 2015954402

Springer Cham Heidelberg New York Dordrecht London

Printed on acid-free paper

Springer International Publishing AG Switzerland is part of Springer Science+Business Media (www.springer.com)

Foreword

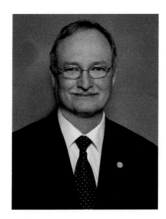

It is my distinct honor and privilege to write the Foreword for Dr. Olivier Courage's book, "Shoulder Arthroscopy: How to Succeed!"

This book is a refreshing addition to the growing list of shoulder arthroscopy texts. But you should know that this book is not like all the others.

I have always thought that the ideal surgical textbook would be one that is clear, concise, and fun to read. Dr. Courage has admirably accomplished all three of these goals with his wonderful book.

Too many surgical textbooks are dull and boring and vague. Looking back to my time in training as an orthopedic resident, I would always try to read about our surgical cases the night before surgery, and oftentimes after reading the surgical techniques in textbooks, I would still not clearly understand how to do the surgery! I recognized at that time the importance of putting technical tips and tricks into a surgical technique description. Yet very few textbooks incorporate technical tips.

However, Dr. Courage not only describes multiple tips and tricks; he has richly illustrated his text with crisp surgical photographs and images that enhance the description of the procedures and principles that he demonstrates.

I have known Oliver Courage for many years, and I have appreciated his talents as a skilled arthroscopic surgeon, a talented educator, and a thought leader in shoulder arthroscopy. His well-deserved election as president of the French Arthroscopy Society is testimony to his leadership skills. Now Dr. Courage demonstrates his expertise in another area, as author of this very engaging book.

Congratulations to my friend Oliver Courage on a job well done!

San Antonio, TX, USA   Stephen S. Burkhart, MD
                                                           July 26, 2015

Foreword

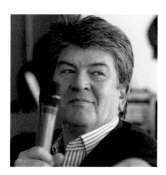

Shoulder arthroscopy is a relatively new and continually evolving surgical technique. It adapts to the different pathologies of the shoulder. It encompasses many therapeutic procedures. It is a technique that requires a long and rigorous learning. Arthroscopic surgery has the particularity that a surgeon does not have to look at their hands, but instead they watch a screen where they see two-dimensional procedures performed three-dimensionally.

Olivier Courage is a particularly experienced shoulder surgeon. He has developed techniques that are specific to him. It is natural that he should want both young people in traineeships and experienced surgeons to benefit from his experience.

Transmission of knowledge is an integral part of a doctor's duties.

Transmission of knowledge is important, but so is its sharing. This is the role of medical publications. It is the companionship that allows the youngest to benefit from the mistakes and successes of the oldest—and for them to do the same later for other young people.

Each surgeon uses (sometimes without even knowing it) technical devices that simplify surgical procedures or facilitate their implementation.

Olivier Courage has taken the time and distance necessary to analyze these procedures, which he has accumulated over his surgical career.

I have learned a great deal from reading his book.

His peers have recognized Olivier Courage as a quality teacherand have elected him president of the *Société Française d'Arthroscopie* [French Society of Arthroscopy].

Olivier Courage has been able to express his principal techniques for facilitating the surgical procedure using simple terms and with a quality illustration. This is where we can see his pedagogical qualities. Everyone will find something to learn in this book whatever their age, whatever their career path.

Boulogne, France   Professor Philippe Hardy

Preface

A skillful boat maneuver is often a narrowly averted disaster. It's the same for shoulder arthroscopy. You should learn to be wary of that which looks simple. This guide is not a technical book; it is a help on how to get yourself out of tricky situations. When we base ourselves on experience, we can reduce the risk of getting into a bad situation.

To make reading more enjoyable, this guide is presented with numerous photos while drawing a parallel with other situations to drive the message home. Some quotes and proverbs are used; they take on their meaning when they are put to the test.

To complete the maritime parallel, bad weather reveals good sailors. It is these situations that allow the fundamentals to emerge. We must quickly develop those saving reflexes. In these cases, the brain needs simple drawers it can open. This is what I have tried to do in this guide.

Happy reading.

Contents

1   **Being in the Right Conditions**   1
    1.1   Avoiding Steam   1
    1.2   Properly Entering the Shoulder   2
    1.3   Avoiding Blood   4

2   **Being Properly Installed**   9
    2.1   Installing the Patient   9
    2.2   The Surgeon's Ergonomy   9

3   **Basic Essentials**   17
    3.1   Stable Image   17
    3.2   Straight Image   17
    3.3   Finding Your Instruments   18

4   **Exploring the Shoulder**   25
    4.1   The Glenohumeral   25
    4.2   The Subacromial Space   28

5   **Tips for the Key Surgeries**   39
    5.1   Before the Surgical Arthroscopy   39
    5.2   The Rotator Cuff   41
    5.3   The Subscapularis   64
    5.4   The Biceps   69
    5.5   Instability and the Arthroscopic Bankart   78

6   **Less Frequent Surgeries**   91
    6.1   The Acromioclavicular   91
    6.2   The Subscapularis Nerve   94

7   **How to Evolve Your Techniques**   97
    7.1   Analyze Your Mistakes, Travel, and Create   97

Conclusion   105

Videos

Video 1: Foundations of shoulder arthroscopy
Video 2: Small tear of the rotator cuff, simplified double row
Video 3: Intermediate tear, speed single bridge
Video 4: Intermediate tear, speed bridge
Video 5: Rotator cuff, how to manage an ear
Video 6: Large tear of the rotator cuff
Video 7: Repair of the subscapularis
Video 8: Biceps tenodesis
Video 9: Bankart and lateral recumbency

Videos on http://extras.springer.com

Being in the Right Conditions

1

1.1 Avoiding Steam

Everything is fine if there is no steam; what to do when it appears and what to do to prevent it?

It is always difficult to eliminate steam.

The steam is caused by the condensation of moisture laden air onto a cold lens.

At sea and in the mountain when fog sets in, things start to go wrong.

A first step is to let air reach the camera inside the cover. For this, we must hold it by the end and leave a "breathing" space (Fig. 1.1).

We can also help patients to reheat by creating a stream of hot air inside the cover.

If this is not enough and we had planned to place a compress inside the cover, we can remove the camera and wipe it. Sometimes it is necessary to change the scope and the cover (Fig. 1.2).

In general, it is too late and even anti-steam products are ineffective (Fig. 1.3).

To prevent steam: be careful when performing the surgical approach (Fig. 1.4).

It must be as small as possible, because the steam comes from the water which is discharged via the posterior approach (Fig. 1.7).

The incision is made with a sharp scalpel, less than 5 mm, and the passage of subcutaneous

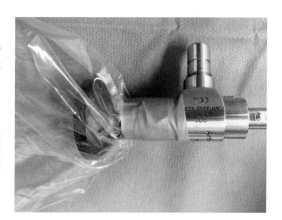

Fig. 1.1

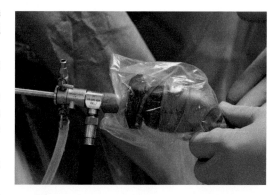

Fig. 1.2

tissue must be performed by rubbing hard with the sharp mandrel. Finally, particular attention should be given to the scope cover sealing by carefully sticking the tape astride (Fig. 1.6).

© Springer International Publishing Switzerland 2015
O. Courage, *Shoulder Arthroscopy: How to Succeed!*, DOI 10.1007/978-3-319-23648-3_1

1

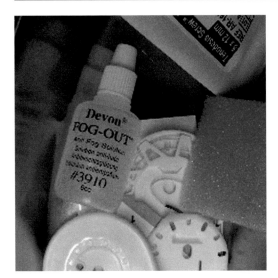

Fig. 1.3

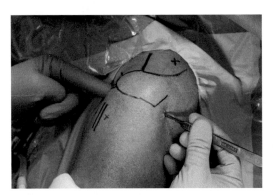

Fig. 1.4

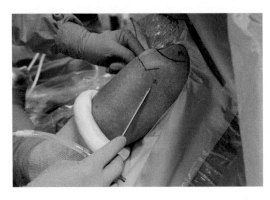

Fig. 1.5

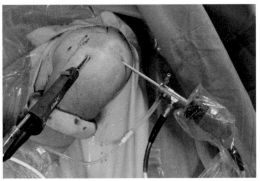

Fig. 1.6

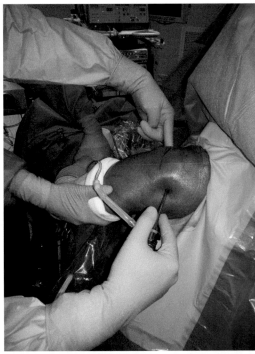

Fig. 1.7

1.2   Properly Entering the Shoulder

It is sometimes difficult to enter the shoulder, without making cartilage lesions.

Sometimes it is not easy to penetrate the shoulder. This is a stressful moment; like an artist, you can't miss your entry.

To enter the capsule, you must decoapt the shoulder but also provide internal rotation; in this way, we stretch the posterior capsule which facilitates the entry of the mandrel (Fig. 1.7).

Moreover, we must aim for the upper section of the articular interline. In this wider area, there is less chance of injuring the cartilage; this is the safety zone (Fig. 1.8).

The point of posterior entry: 2 cm downward and inward from the posterior angle of the acromion is sometimes difficult to palpate. It can be reliably found with the thumb and index finger. This way of palpating that you see in the image is very useful in obese patients. This is the most important point to draw before starting (Fig. 1.9).

The axis is also very important; we must aim for the coracoid (we often go too far outside). Sometimes it is also because we have not taken the time to appreciate the shoulder's size. Between a rugby player and a small hairdresser, the difference in joint size can be twofold. A good way of appreciating this size is to draw the various bony structures. This is a kind of reconnaissance, before the procedure (Fig. 1.10).

Once this axis is felt well inside the space, we can draw other bony landmarks in order: the acromioclavicular joint, the lateral edge of the acromion, the spine of the scapula, the clavicle with its anterior and posterior edge, the coracoid, and finally the coracoacromial ligament (Fig. 1.11).

We end with the approaches that we are likely to perform.

If a surgery on the biceps is planned, the groove will be drawn. It is often difficult to palpate and we often place it too far outside. In neutral rotation, it is in the middle, well in the direction of the biceps (Fig. 1.12).

To enter the shoulder once you are safely inside the safety zone and if the capsule is difficult to pass, you can use a pointed mandrel, and with a firm gesture (like in karate), enter the capsule and synovium (Fig. 1.13).

Before positioning the lens, we turn on the water, and we look to see whether the pump is running. Once we have verified this, the mandrel is removed and it is confirmed by the return of water. This is a time-saver, and it avoids meandering around the soft parts (Fig. 1.14).

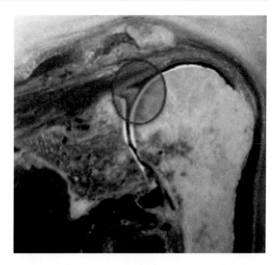

Fig. 1.8

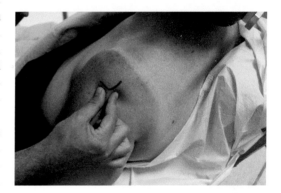

Fig. 1.9

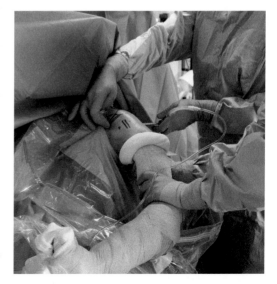

Fig. 1.10

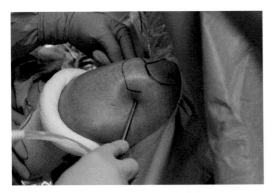

Fig. 1.11

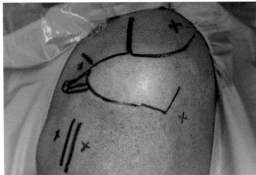

Fig. 1.13

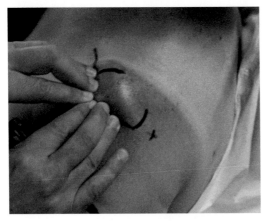

Fig. 1.12

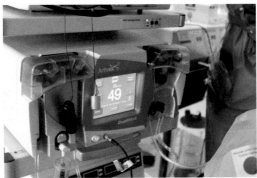

Fig. 1.14

1.3   Avoiding Blood

I have blood, the image is all red…

When the shoulder is red and the joint looks like the Japanese flag, don't lose your cool (Figs. 1.15 and 1.16).

There are several parameters on which to act. Before anything else, check that nothing is preventing water circulation: tap closed, tube angled, and tube clamp too tight (Fig. 1.17).

We must bear in mind this drawing that compares the shoulder to a ball.

By acting on the set of parameters, it is possible to recuperate a good vision. The size of the surgical approaches is again fundamental here, the smallest possible! (Fig. 1.18)

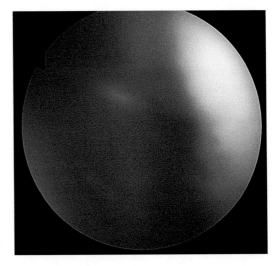

Fig. 1.15

The suction of the shaver must be weak and only used when we require it. Blood pressure will be as low as possible (less than 100 mmHg) (Fig. 1.19).

The pump pressure is permanently set; the lowest for properly seeing without over-inflating the shoulder. The circulating nurse must keep an eye on this (Fig. 1.20).

One can also use a remote control oneself for the pump which allows the pressure to be instantaneously adapted (Figs. 1.21 and 1.22).

Do not panic if the shoulder inflates; there are never any neurological complications as the liquid diffuses without risk of compression. On the other hand, the surgery will be technically more difficult on these big shoulders. You must always try to do a hemostasis (Figs. 1.23 and 1.24).

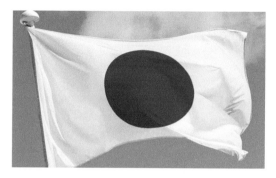

Fig. 1.16

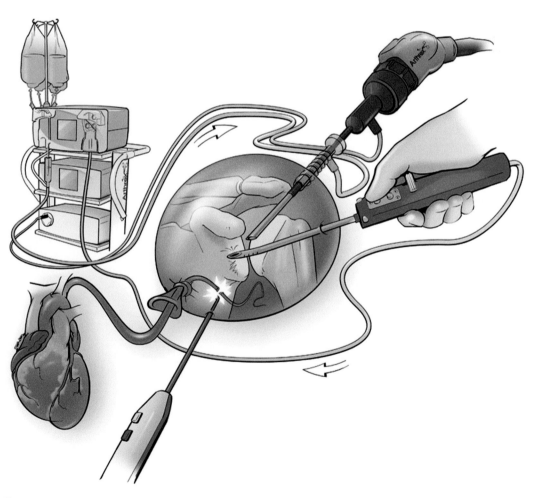

Fig. 1.17

Finally, a water leak creates a current and decreases the pressure (Bernoulli's theorem), the shoulder collapses, and vision is poor. Rather than using a finger to seal, a compress will have the same effect. It also prevents the assistants getting drenched (Figs. 1.25 and 1.26).

You must continually act on these different parameters to maintain a good vision. You must never fall behind, and each team member must be concentrated on the subject. This is one of the major keys to success in shoulder arthroscopy!

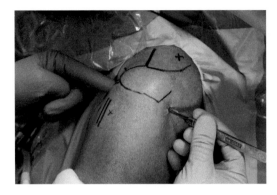

Fig. 1.18

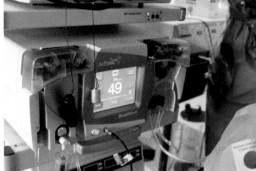

Fig. 1.20

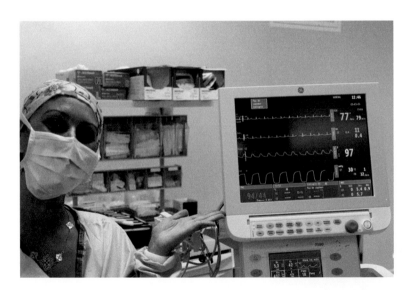

Fig. 1.19

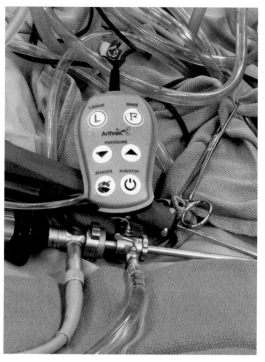

Fig. 1.21

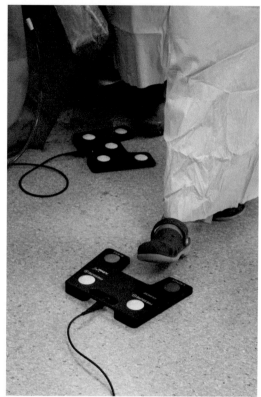

Fig. 1.22

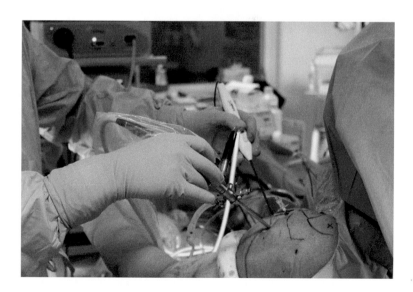

Fig. 1.23

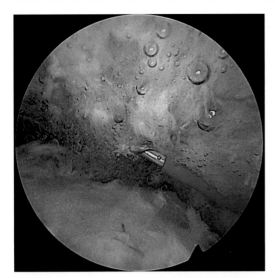

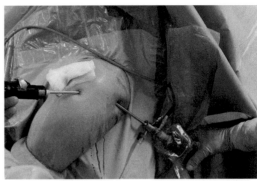

Fig. 1.26

Fig. 1.24

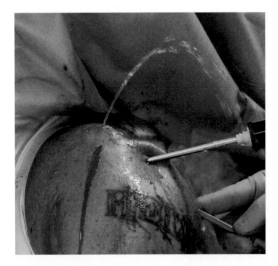

Fig. 1.25

Being Properly Installed

2.1 Installing the Patient

> To work inside the subacromial space, we are sometimes bothered by the table which prevents the scope being medialized.

The easiest in this case for a cuff is to change the surgical approach for a lateral approach. We shall see this in the cuff chapter. As in any surgery, the installation is essential (Fig. 2.1).

Care must be taken to have an unobstructed shoulder. This is always the case in lateral recumbency (Figs. 2.1 and 2.3).

Incidentally, it is very important to check the pressure points oneself. We must anticipate the risks of lesion. This installation is checked before surgery, but it must also be checked during surgery either by the circulating nurse or by the anesthetist. The endotracheal tube is preferably placed at the opposite side of the operated shoulder (Figs. 2.4 and 2.5).

Be careful during surgeries; we tend to "pull" to decoapt and the cervical spine of the patient can be very overworked.

The installation of the arm must be carefully performed, and the support points must be protected. We must consider the different positions that will be required for exploration and the different procedures to be performed. To avoid any difficulties in case of problems, be sure to use devices in keeping with the standards (Figs. 2.6 and 2.7).

2.2 The Surgeon's Ergonomy

> Ergonomics aims to adapt a system to its user, so that the latter operates with maximum efficiency, satisfaction, and well-being, with a reduced adaptation phase.

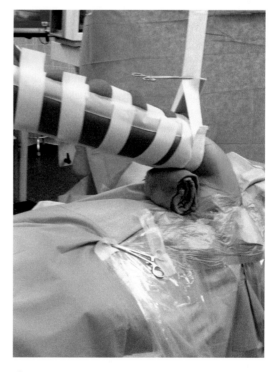

Fig. 2.1

O. Courage, *Shoulder Arthroscopy: How to Succeed!*, DOI 10.1007/978-3-319-23648-3_2

We must not only think of the patient; we must also think of ourselves and our team.

Install the screens opposite to you at eye level (Fig. 2.8).

We must try to place the screens according to the procedure to be performed. For example, in case of biceps tenodesis, if there are two screens, the second one will be placed near the patient's head (Fig. 2.9).

It is preferable to use pedals for shaving the patient; that means you don't have to take your eyes off the screen during usage. A handheld remote control for the Arthropump allows us to work in optimal viewing conditions (Figs. 2.10 and 2.11).

We must check the height of the table to save our shoulders (Fig. 2.12).

On the instrumentalist's table, you must have the minimal instruments laid out in order and available to hand (on a bridge table or on the patient): the shaver, the lens, and the electrode (Figs. 2.13 and 2.14).

Finally, the use of an articulated arm also frees the assistant and allows the rotation, ABD, and ADD of the limb to be fixed, which is sometimes useful for positioning the implants. The decoaptation can also be improved; the liquid collection bag can be cited here (Fig. 2.15).

Also, for safety reasons, it is good to separate the water from the electricity and make sure that the Arthropump pockets are away from the spine (Fig. 2.16).

Finally, a simple compress on a surgical approach avoids the assistant getting wet or

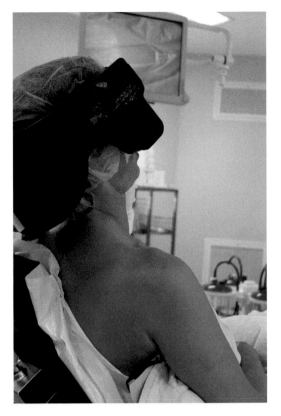

Fig. 2.2

having to crouch down to avoid getting drenched. Moreover the intra-articular vision will be improved by avoiding a water stream which decreases intra-articular pressure (Figs. 2.17 and 2.18).

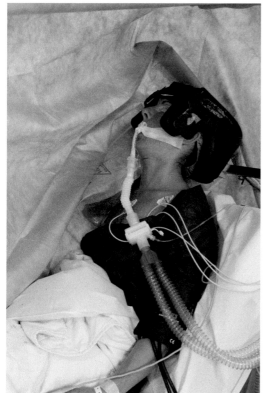

Fig. 2.3

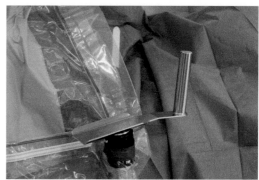

Fig. 2.5

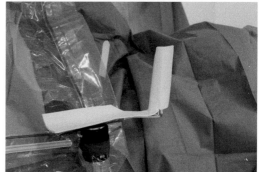

Fig. 2.6

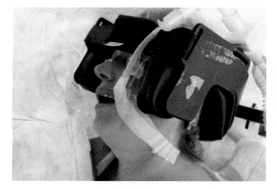

Fig. 2.4

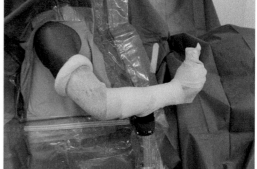

Fig. 2.7

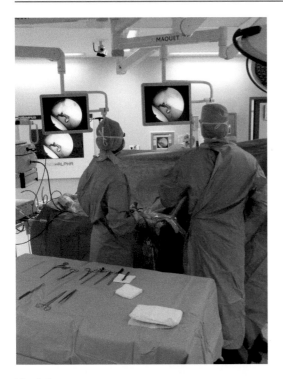

Fig. 2.8

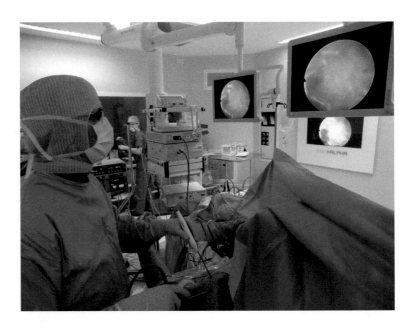

Fig. 2.9

Fig. 2.10

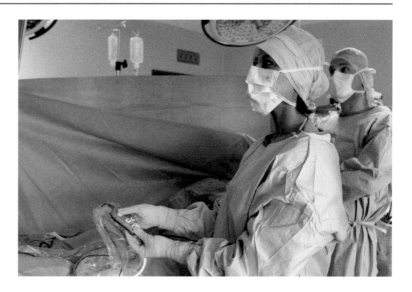

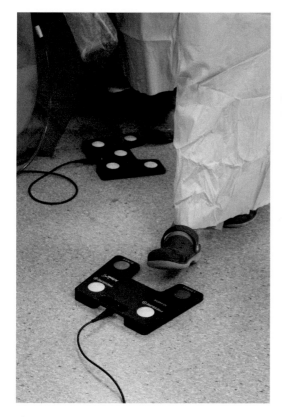

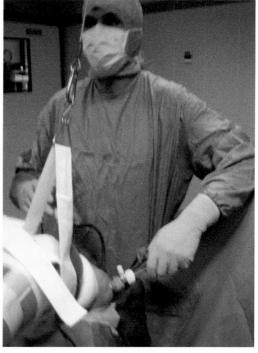

Fig. 2.12

Fig. 2.11

Fig. 2.13

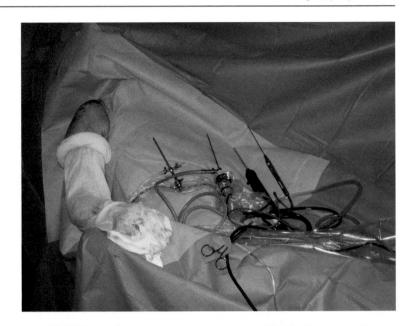

Fig. 2.14

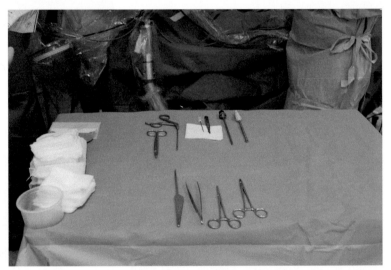

Fig. 2.15

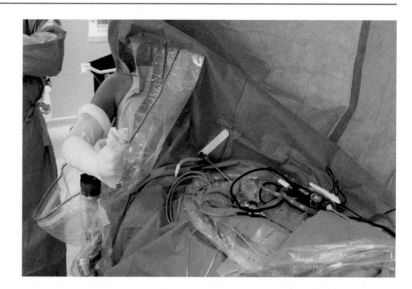

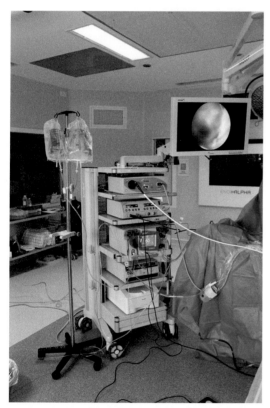

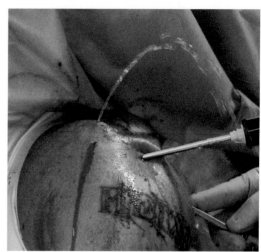

Fig. 2.17

Fig. 2.16

Fig. 2.18

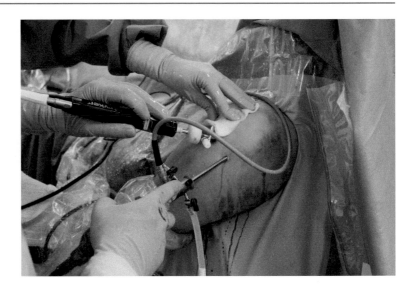

Basic Essentials

3

3.1 Stable Image

There is nothing more tedious than an unstable image for the surgeon but also for the assistants and observers (Fig. 3.1).

There is a good technique for holding the camera. As in billiards, the fingers form a tripod that stabilizes the rod. This also avoids putting the scope too close to the area affected by the surgery. Taking a step back makes things easier (as in life) (Fig. 3.2).

This way of holding the camera also avoids inconvenient removals of the scope, particularly during the anterior exploration of the shoulder.

Moreover, this way of holding the scope tells us (without having to look at our hands) the position of the optical fiber and thus the scope's orientation (Fig. 3.2).

It is preferable to have large hands, but everyone finds the position that suits them.

3.2 Straight Image

To operate properly, it is essential to always keep an image properly straight.

When filming our holidays, the camera always remains vertical, even by boat; the horizon is a landmark for the view. It is the same for our shoulder surgeries. You must not tilt your head during the operation; it is the image that must stay straight. This requires benchmarks.

In half-sitting position, the tendon of the sub-scapularis is the horizon of the shoulder. The challenge is to keep this benchmark even when using the strong oblique of the scope. The scope turns but not the camera, for this a simple way is to always have the cable of the camera vertical, or

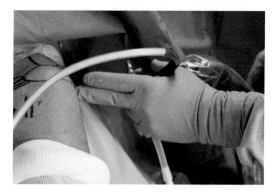

Fig. 3.1

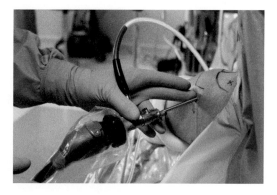

Fig. 3.2

© Springer International Publishing Switzerland 2015
O. Courage, *Shoulder Arthroscopy: How to Succeed!*, DOI 10.1007/978-3-319-23648-3_3

rather it must be the bisector of the arm and the chest (Fig. 3.4).

When we are in the subacromial space, we do not have this benchmark that is the subscapularis tendon. In half-sitting position, the acromion must be horizontal. Another approach to take is to see our display instruments in the screen with the same angle as we look at our hands (Fig. 3.5).

It is a sort of reality TV. You must see the same thing on the screen as when you are looking at the instruments directly. This approach accelerates learning; in fact the brain has benchmarks. Procedural coordination is facilitated by this coherence. Of course in lateral recumbency, the glenoid will be horizontal (Fig. 3.6).

3.3   Finding Your Instruments

I cannot easily find my instruments in the shoulder!

The most common mistake is to search for them while watching the screen. We're still watching too much TV!

To properly triangulate, we must watch our hands on a regular basis. The right choice of surgical approaches is important. We must know how to use our index finger as our natural viewfinder. So for finding the subacromial space, place your index finger on the acromion to locate yourself (Figs. 3.7 and 3.8).

Then, once the second surgical approach has been performed, we must find the contact between the mandrel of the scope and the shaver.

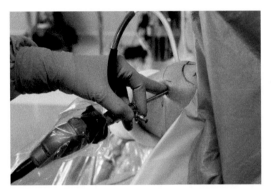

Fig. 3.3

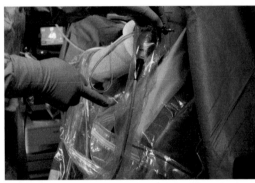

Fig. 3.4

Fig. 3.5

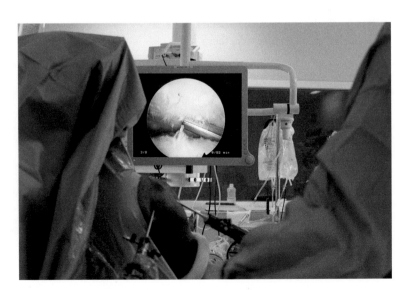

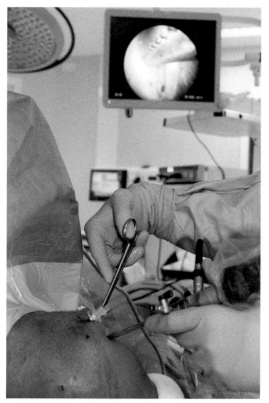

Fig. 3.6

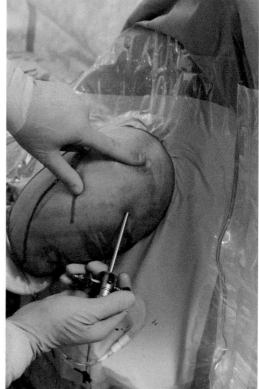

Fig. 3.7

Proceeding this way before placing the lens will avoid unnecessary shocks (Fig. 3.9).

By doing so, we feel the contact between the tip of the mandrel and the tip of the shaver; you have to concentrate to feel this "triangulation." For a cuff, there is a true triangulation; it is like a moped handlebar (Figs. 3.10, 3.11, and 3.12).

In terms of instability, it is rather like a scooter (Figs. 3.13 and 3.14).

Sometimes when an instrument is lost, it is best to remove the lens in order to feel the contact again and then put it back. This (conservative)

way of proceeding limits the risks of damaging the lenses. When we lose sight of the instrument, the most common mistake is to keep your eyes fixed on the screen and "shuffle around" to find it again. In fact good sense in this case dictates that you take your eyes off the screen and look at your hands; then you align the triangle as necessary with the help of your "index finger, natural view-finder," and then you find that you've saved time (Figs. 3.15, 3.16, and 3.17).

Before these first surgeries, a mock training is recommended (Figs. 3.18 and 3.19).

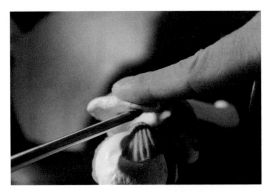

Fig. 3.8

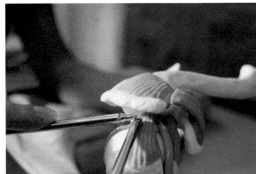

Fig. 3.9

Fig. 3.10

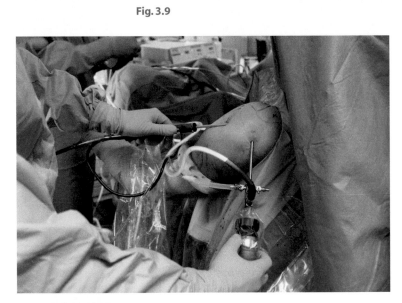

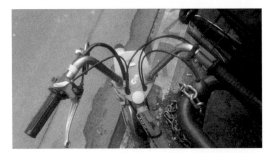

Fig. 3.11

Fig. 3.12

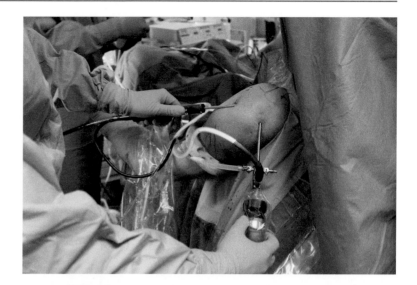

Fig. 3.13

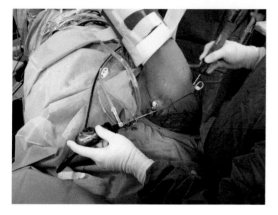

Fig. 3.14

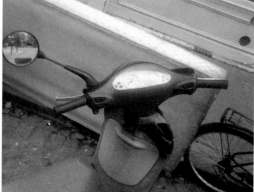

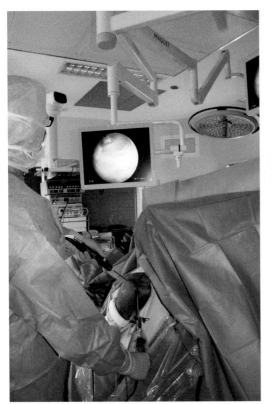

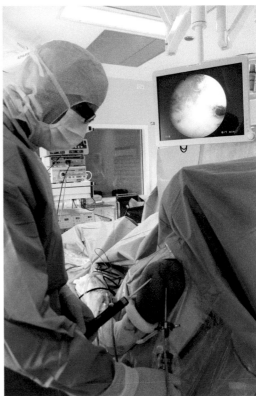

Fig. 3.15   **Fig. 3.16**

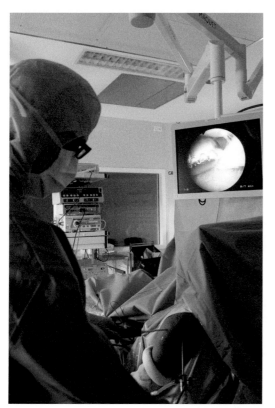

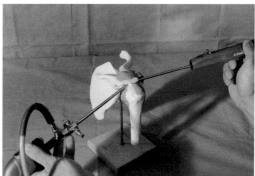

Fig. 3.18

Fig. 3.17

Fig. 3.19

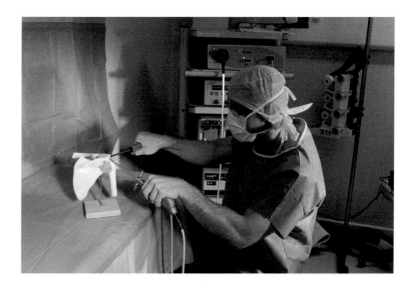

Exploring the Shoulder

4

4.1 The Glenohumeral

As with any surgery, there must be order.
We have ten points to check.

The safety zone is the anterior triangle formed by the glenoid, the biceps, and the tendon of the subscapularis.

When starting to explore the shoulder through this zone, we are not going to run the risk of exiting the shoulder. Any exiting is a waste of time and an additional steam risk.

We must use the forward oblique of the scope (Fig. 4.1).

Point 1

The condition of the glenoid cartilage (to be mentioned in the CRO), because it can explain pain. The umbilical central zone is physiological; it serves as a bare spot for measuring glenoid bone defects (Fig. 4.2).

Point 2

The cartilage of the humeral head and a possible notch (Fig. 4.3).

Point 3

For the subscapularis, take your time and place the shoulder in internal rotation by directing the scope outward and using the probe to search for hidden damage (Figs. 4.4, 4.5, 4.6, and 4.7).

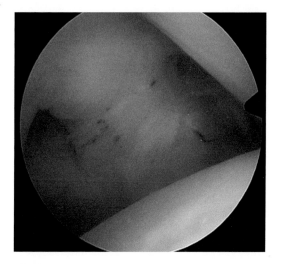

Fig. 4.1

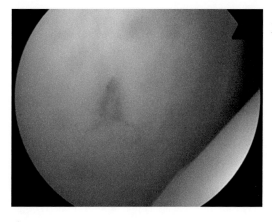

Fig. 4.2

© Springer International Publishing Switzerland 2015
O. Courage, *Shoulder Arthroscopy: How to Succeed!*, DOI 10.1007/978-3-319-23648-3_4

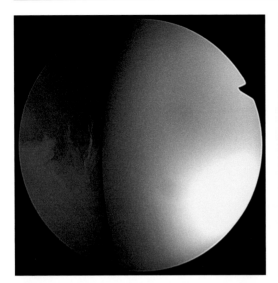

Fig. 4.3

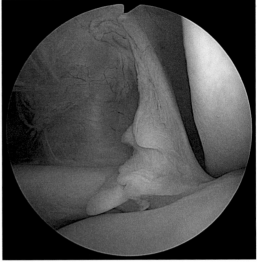

Fig. 4.5

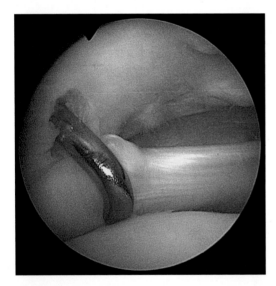

Fig. 4.4

Point 4
The biceps and the groove with the coracohumeral ligament will be explored with the help of the probe and by rotation. A dynamic exploration can be performed in the search for an instability. Placing the shoulder in forward flexion can also generate this space (Figs. 4.8, 4.9, 4.10, and 4.11).

Point 5
The SLAP is searched by placing the strong oblique upward, and the probe is essential for diagnosis (Figs. 4.12 and 4.13).

Point 6
We continue downward, and the forward oblique of the scope is oriented inward; the probe is also recommended for the labrum (Fig. 4.14).

Point 7
Then we explore the inferior recess without forgetting the humeral lateral in search of an HAGL; we sometimes find surprises in this recess, such as loose bodies. We then return the scope toward the front into the safety zone (Figs. 4.15 and 4.16).

Point 8
The arm is then abducted to properly clear the insertion of the supraspinatus, and the forward oblique of the scope is oriented outward (Figs. 4.17 and 4.18).

Point 9
Then we continue the exploration behind toward the infraspinatus; the bald area serves as a benchmark (Fig. 4.19).

Fig. 4.6

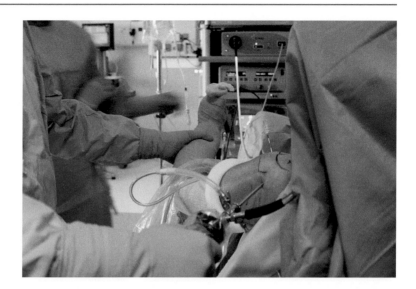

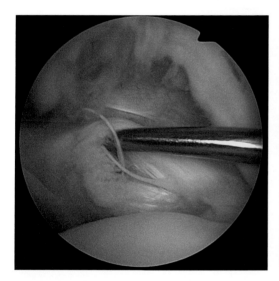

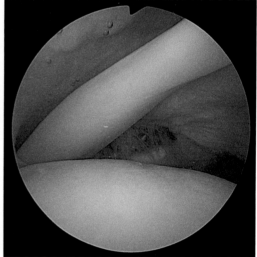

Fig. 4.7   **Fig. 4.8**

Point 10

We then visualize the anterior labrum. At this moment, the risk of exiting is significant (Fig. 4.20).

Exploration is systematic, and these **ten points help us not to forget anything.**

We must also bear in mind our clinical examination and investigations in the search for a lesion. For example, an O'Brien maneuver or a sub-dislocated biceps with MRI will make us explore the biceps and its grooves very carefully.

Similarly, an MRI arthrography which leads us to suspect a subscapularis lesion will make us particularly careful when exploring this latter (Figs. 4.21 and 4.22).

An exploration by anterior approach in case of shoulder instability is sometimes recommended. To accomplish this, the Wissinger rod is required. The camera's orientation can cause a problem; having the cable upward in this reversed exploration facilitates the orientation. We see this way of proceeding in the instability.

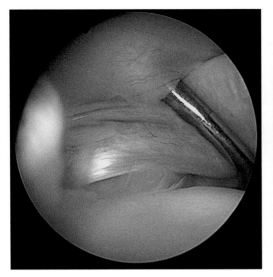

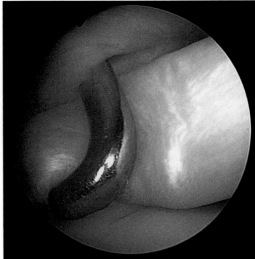

Fig. 4.9   Fig. 4.10

Fig. 4.11

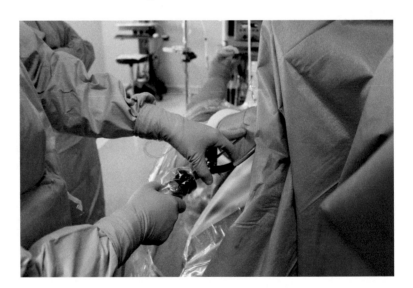

The difficulty in this exploration is to properly coordinate the usage of the foreward oblique with the mobilization of the arm (Figs. 4.23 and 4.24).

4.2   The Subacromial Space

My vision in the subacromial bursa is not good.

To be sure to be in the right space, you must use your natural viewfinder: your index finger is subacromially placed, and then you use the scope with its mandrel of the posterior approach (the lens is removed to protect it). You must then pass under the posterior edge toward the pulp of your index finger (as if to scratch your finger). Some oscillations upward allow the acromion to be clearly felt, and beforehand, a projection indicates that we are on the coracoacromial ligament (Figs. 4.25 and 4.26).

The lateral approach must be sufficiently low. It is often recommended to perform it 2 cm below the lateral edge of the acromion. However, at 3 cm, it is more comfortable because the

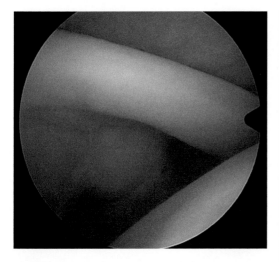

Fig. 4.12

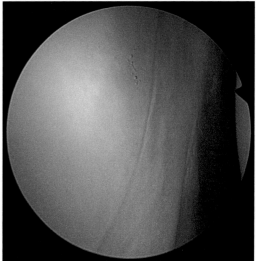

Fig. 4.14

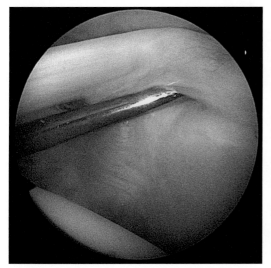

Fig. 4.13

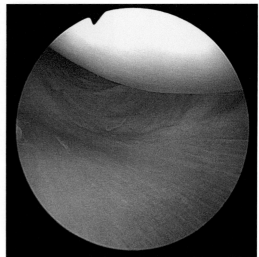

Fig. 4.15

instrument works tangentially to the space and not in "nose dive." Before placing the lenses, we must put the end of the mandrel and the end of the shaver into contact. It saves time and scopes! (Figs. 4.27 and 4.28)

The hand holding the camera should also be lowered to improve the field of vision.

The bad reflex for seeing better is to raise your hands (as if you were going on tiptoe). In this case, the scope flattens against the tissues and vision is poor. To see well, you must lower it and

remember the design of the swing (Figs. 4.29, 4.30, 4.31, and 4.32).

Once you can see the shaver in the bursa, you must begin the bursectomy from the front and the outside (shaver teeth upward). It takes patience to clean the bursa; consider doing it laterally. This lateral learning is very useful for cuff repair techniques by cerclage. This is to be done at the beginning without cannula; this makes it easier. Otherwise once the cannula is in place, this lateral bursectomy is more difficult to achieve; it

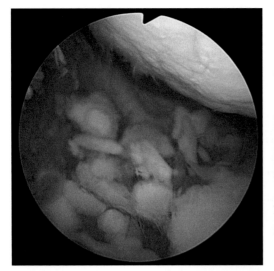

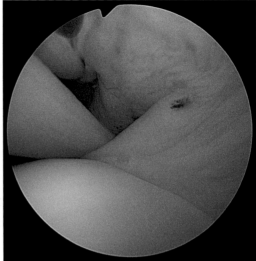

Fig. 4.16

Fig. 4.17

Fig. 4.18

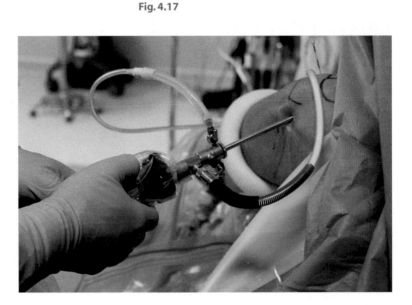

turns into a canulectomy (Figs. 4.33, 4.34, 4.35, and 4.36).

The bursectomy is a critical stage, as in the event of inflammation of the bursa, it is without doubt the most important procedure for pain reduction. Moreover, it is easier to perform in case of lesion of the cuff or calcification. You should never save time on cleaning; you will soon regret it.

A good worker is recognized by the cleanliness of their work site!

We can then proceed to the acromion.

You must use the obliquity of the scope and not forget to direct it upward while always keeping the image straight. Think of the scope as an eye that you need to move in all directions.

If the scope is properly oriented, the camera remains vertical. The arthroscope is the eye, and the cold light cable is the braid (Fig. 4.37).

As shown in photo 15, we have used the obliquity of the scope, but the image remains straight. The acromion that we see must be dissected before using an electric probe or sheathed knife (Figs. 4.38, 4.39, 4.40, and 4.41).

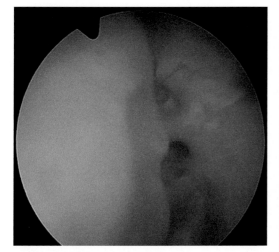

Fig. 4.19

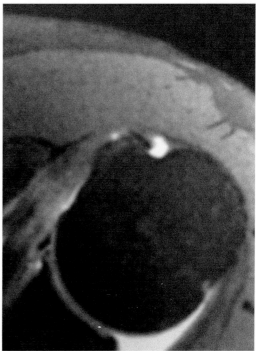

Fig. 4.21

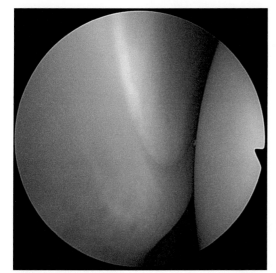

Fig. 4.20

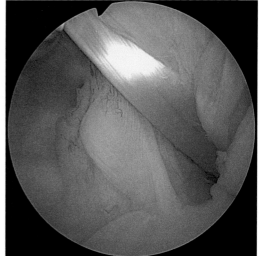

Fig. 4.22

It is important to perform this dissection beforehand; otherwise we may leave an osteophyte there. By being flush with the bone and meticulous during this stage, we avoid the branch of the acromioclavicular chest. This stage also prevents bleeding which would render the following steps difficult.

For acromioplasty, it is recommended to start with the anterolateral angle of the acromion. This is the most difficult place to reach and to see, but this is where the conflict is situated. Moreover, if we start the acromioplasty in the middle, there is a risk of making a "Roman tile" (which is also bad luck for the patient) (Figs. 4.42, 4.43, 4.44, and 4.45).

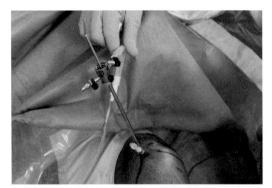

Fig. 4.23

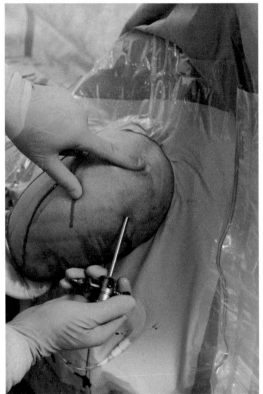

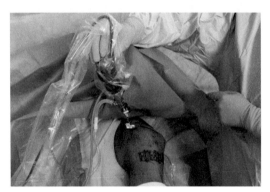

Fig. 4.24

Fig. 4.25

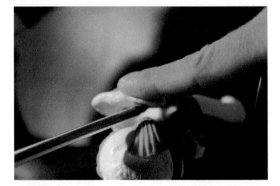

Fig. 4.26

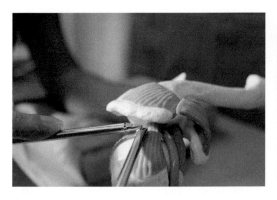

Fig. 4.27

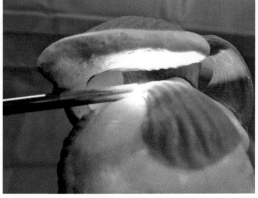

Fig. 4.29

Fig. 4.28

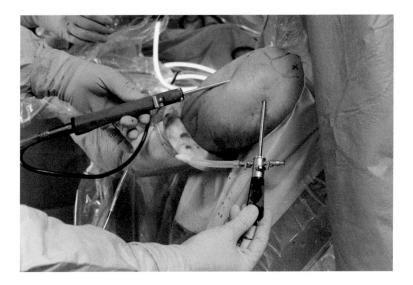

Fig. 4.30

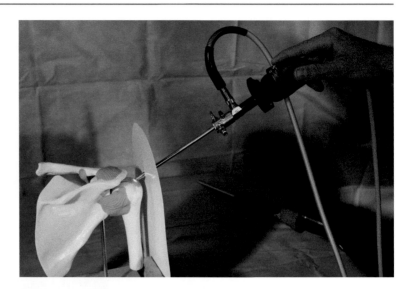

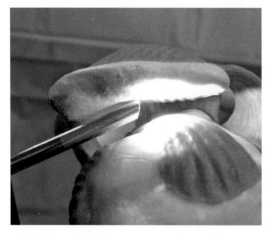

Fig. 4.31

Fig. 4.32

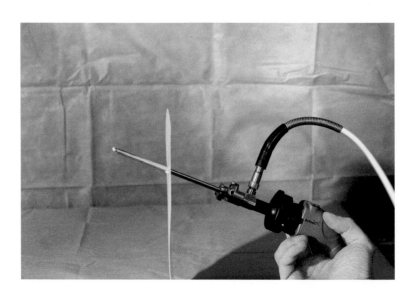

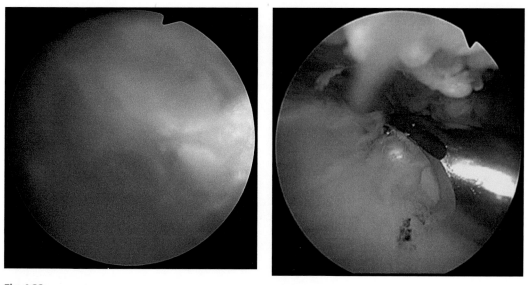

Fig. 4.33

Fig. 4.35

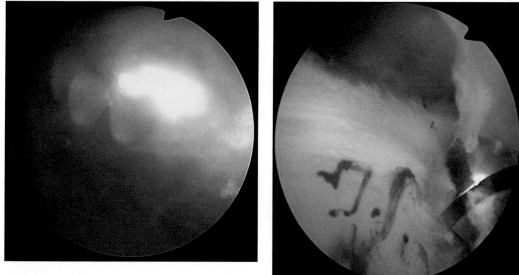

Fig. 4.34

Fig. 4.36

Fig. 4.37

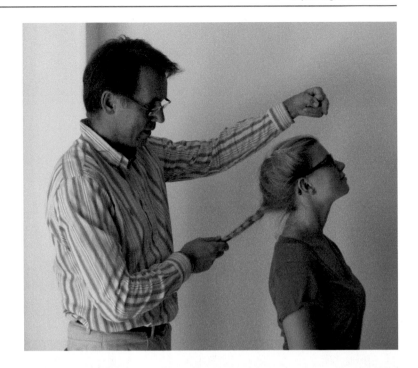

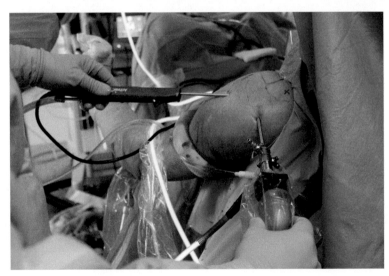

Fig. 4.38

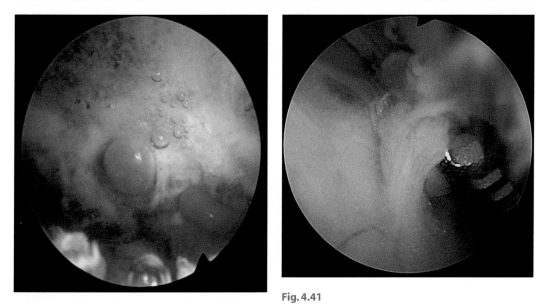

Fig. 4.39

Fig. 4.41

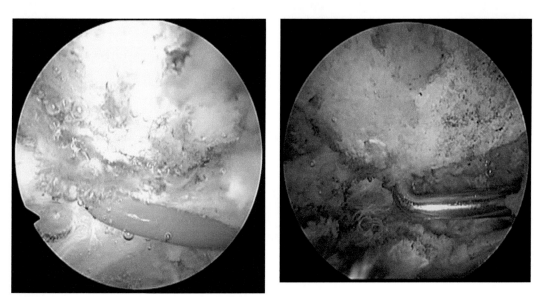

Fig. 4.40

Fig. 4.42

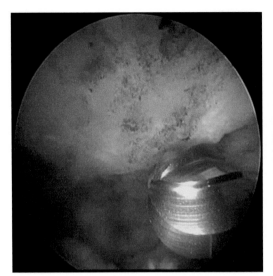

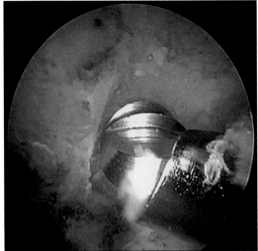

Fig. 4.45

Fig. 4.43

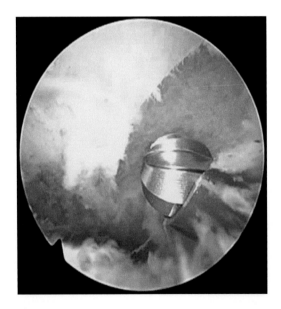

Fig. 4.44

Tips for the Key Surgeries

5

5.1 Before the Surgical Arthroscopy

We will now move onto the surgical arthroscopy. When seen on videos or performed by trained surgeons, it appears easy. But as always, beware of what appears simple.

Windsurfing, kitesurfing, music, tennis, and golf are examples of activities that when performed by regulars appear simple, but behind this simplicity hides a great deal of work. Surgery is no exception to this rule. Before completing this step, you must train with modesty.

The commonest blockage is the execution of arthroscopic knots.

If they slide, the simplest is the Laurent Lafosse knot (easy knot!); it never sticks, and you must choose the traction strand or post on which the suture is sliding (Figs. 5.1, 5.2, and 5.3).

It begins with three half hitches in the same direction, keeping the post properly taut.

The fourth half hitch is then reversed, and the fifth is made like the first three (Figs. 5.4 and 5.5).

Note that the knot must go beyond the knot for the locking.

But beware; when the sutures do not slide, they must be done half hitch by half hitch.

You must not perform your first knots on a patient but on a test bench.

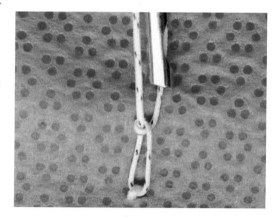

Fig. 5.1

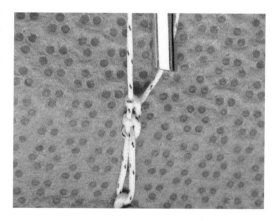

Fig. 5.2

© Springer International Publishing Switzerland 2015
O. Courage, *Shoulder Arthroscopy: How to Succeed!*, DOI 10.1007/978-3-319-23648-3_5

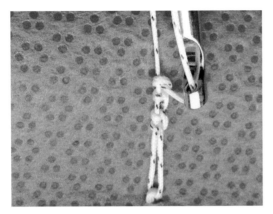

Fig. 5.3

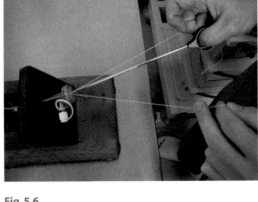

Fig. 5.6

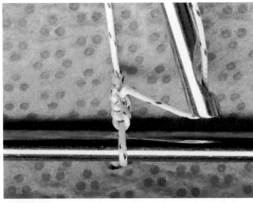

Fig. 5.4

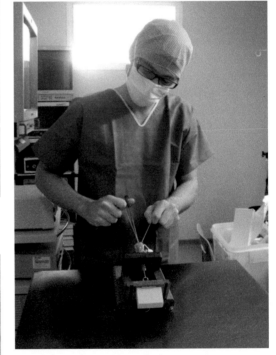

Fig. 5.7

Fig. 5.5

This procedure requiring both hands and the handling of sutures requires some learning. Take a good look at the photo that shows how to block

the sutures with your fingers (Figs. 5.6, 5.7, and 5.8).

Note that during this phase, both hands are occupied, so you need to have trained the instrumentalist on how to operate the camera.

Ballet on three hands and learning: while we're doing the knot, the instrumentalist is doing the filming!

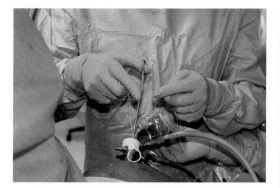

Fig. 5.8

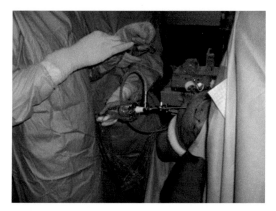

Fig. 5.9

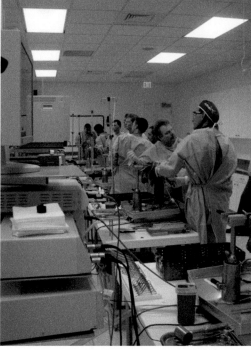

Fig. 5.10

5.2 The Rotator Cuff

Repair of the rotator cuff is the queen of all surgical arthroscopy indications.

It is sometimes difficult to see the rotator cuff and especially to assess its size and shape.

Courses on corpses are useful steps before moving onto our patients (Figs. 5.9 and 5.10).

Mentoring has an important place in this learning phase (Fig. 5.11).

You must always think about these patients of the learning curve and always give oneself a solution to fall back on in case of problem, or beyond a certain surgery time. The surgical approach for a cuff is performed by using what we have seen during the arthroscopy. In general, it is sufficient to enlarge the instrumental approach on both sides, in order to finish with open procedure. The patient won't blame you if they have been forewarned, and that also allows them to understand the reason for the difficulty. In passing a palpation of the acromioplasty enables us to progress (Fig. 5.12).

The scope must overhang the lesion. Like for drawing a country on a map, the satellite must be plumb. Changing the posterior optical portal for a lateral portal also allows an improved assessment of the posterior edge of the cuff, which is often delaminated. Similarly, a tear considered to be C-shaped when we leave the scope by posterior approach is in fact V-shaped, when the scope is laterally placed.

The discovery of the tear is performed in intra-articular (Fig. 5.13); we thus confirm the

Fig. 5.11

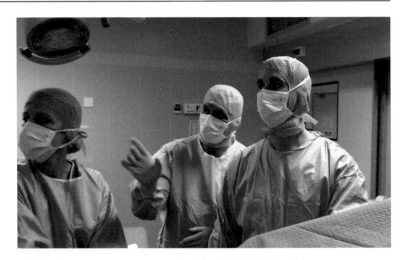

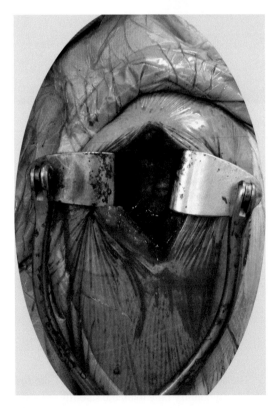

Fig. 5.12

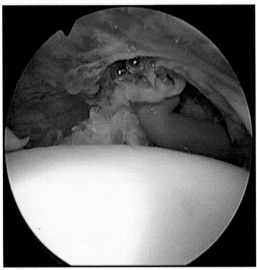

Fig. 5.13

transfixing character; the scope is then subacromially passed after the bursectomy (Figs. 5.14 and 5.15).

This vision is misleading. The scope is not above the lesion; very often, this gives an overly optimistic vision. Too often we have the impression of a C-shaped tear that will be easy to close, and in addition, we do not see the posterior edge of the tear clearly.

Like a satellite over a country, the scope must be laterally moved (Figs. 5.16, 5.17, and 5.18).

Indeed, the vision of the tear that we see on the screen is actually a representation. This is a projection of a rotator cuff, which is a sphere portion, onto a flat screen.

Remaining with the posterior approach, we would undoubtedly not see the delamination of the posterior layer. In this case, due to ignorance, we run a significant risk of only closing the superficial layer.

Fig. 5.14

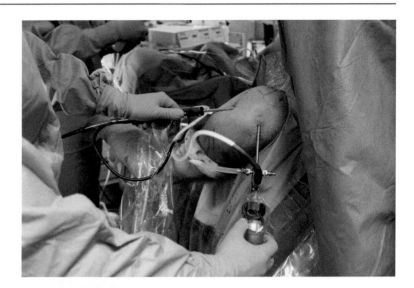

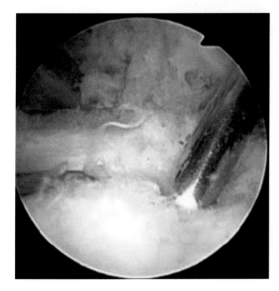

Fig. 5.15

Despite the analysis of the shape, certain tears are sometimes difficult to close.

The drawings are always a bit theoretical; don't neglect wear, which is why to close some tears trade-offs must often be made. The key is to always close without tension. For this, dynamic analysis is fundamental; it is performed using a grasper. It is by making these dynamic maneuvers that we understand the tear's shape. So it consists of an L-shaped tear when the gentle traction on an angle allows the tear to be completely closed without tension. Without this dynamic

analysis, it is impossible to diagnose these L-shaped tears. That is why they are never described by radiologists (Figs. 5.19, 5.20, 5.21, and 5.22).

Theory: the C, the V, the L, practice, etc. wear and its trade-offs

Whatever the technique used, the next stage is the acromioplasty and the section of the LAC, if it is necessary.

Note If the tear is not repairable, it is better to leave the LAC in place; it sometimes allows the patient an anterior elevation. Like a golf swing, it is the kinetic energy at the point of contact: the lesser tuberosity of the humerus that allows elevation.

The next stage is not very difficult; it consists of freshening the tuberosity. It is easier to do it without cannula. If the bone is fragile, we can turn the round burr upside down. Otherwise, in case of sclerotic bone, we can be helped by a curette or punch micro fractures to be sure to have healthy living bone, which will improve healing thanks to stem cells.

It is sometimes difficult to position the implants after having freshened the tuberosity.

For your first cuff repairs, it is better to perform a single-row technique. We can quickly perform double points combining vertical and horizontal points so that the implants are mounted in double suture (Figs. 5.23 and 5.24).

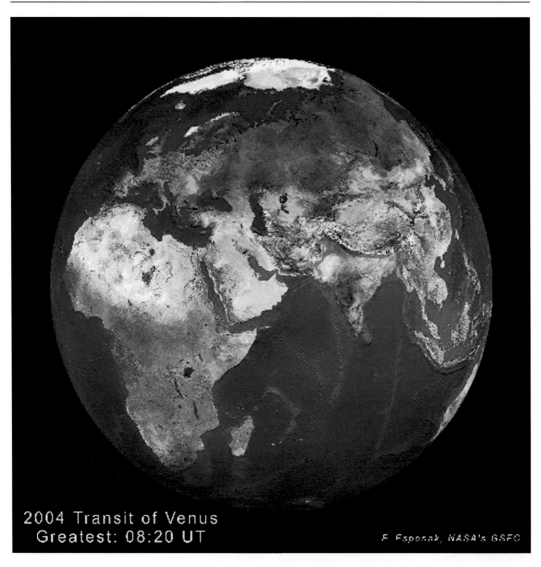

Fig. 5.16

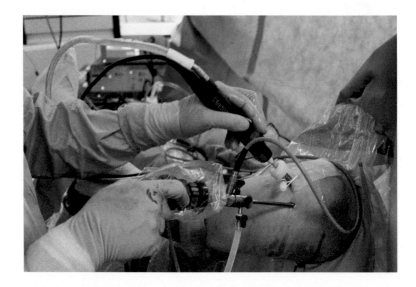

Fig. 5.17

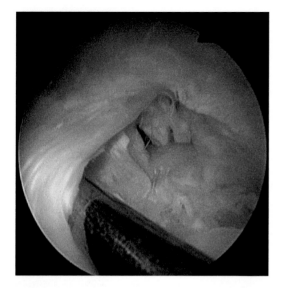

Fig. 5.18

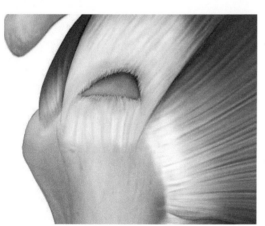

Fig. 5.19

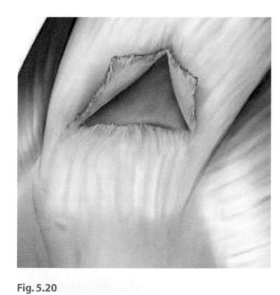

Fig. 5.20

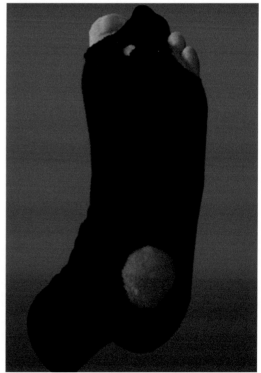

Fig. 5.21

Fig. 5.22

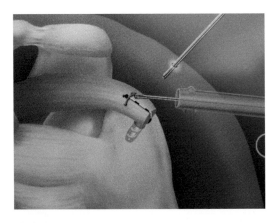

Fig. 5.23

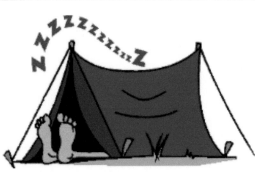

Fig. 5.26

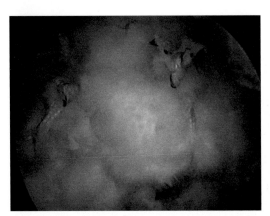

Fig. 5.24

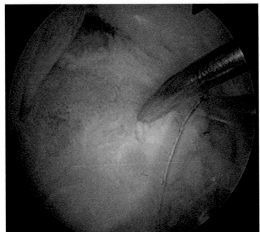

Fig. 5.27

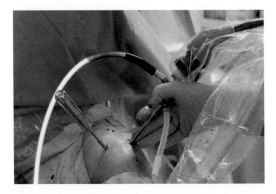

Fig. 5.25

For the single row, we must put the implant in the middle of the tuberosity. Placing the arm in light adduction and directing the scope downward facilitate the exposure (Fig. 5.25).

To locate oneself, use a long OL needle. It also helps to choose the incidence of 45°, like a tent peg. To save time, if we are using a cannula, it is possible to use it as a viewfinder to find the correct position of the implant. We must look at our hands rather than fight while watching TV (Figs. 5.26, 5.27, and 5.28).

You can end up mistaking the wire when catching the sutures and even removing them from the implant.

Before making a suture, you need a short time of concentration (especially when it is late).

A good rule of thumb is to see three elements: tear, implant and sutures, and the cannula or the opening. Do not pull too fast if you do not see clearly (Fig. 5.29).

A suture already placed in the cuff can be identified by a small forceps. Do not pull on a

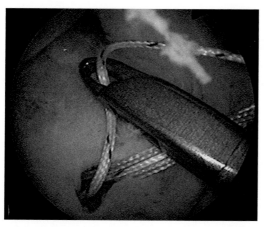

Fig. 5.28

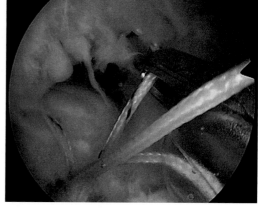

Fig. 5.31

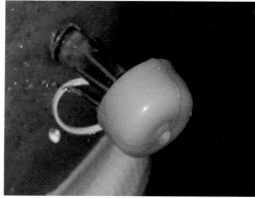

Fig. 5.32

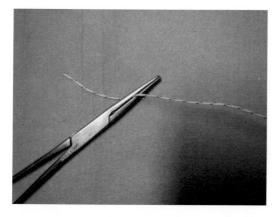

Fig. 5.29

Fig. 5.30

blocked suture in the cannula or in the valves of the scope; do not force and once again remember to look at your hands. To see and avoid mistakes, we must know how to take care of the preparation and, when you decide to pull out a suture, how to control the implant with the scope (Figs. 5.30, 5.31, and 5.32).

With forceps, tissue clamping is sometimes insufficient, but with the curved needle (Banana Lasso® Arthrex), we decide on the width of the tissue to be loaded (Figs. 5.33, 5.34, 5.35, and 5.36).

You must do it simply and pass the sutures one by one; this prevents them from becoming tangled. The Banana Lasso must be used as follows (Figs. 5.37, 5.38, 5.39, and 5.40).

On a small distal supraspinatus tear:

- You use the upper surgical approach of Neviaser; do not hesitate to use the index finger of the other hand as a viewfinder to find the direction and the correct space.
- Then you have to "mimic" the procedure above the cuff to accustom your hand to the correct direction.
- You can transfix the cuff at the determined distance.
- Then after the suture, you can capture the relay in the cannula. A large tissue clamping is

the guarantee of a good coverage of the insertion zone.

Once the suture or the relay is passed, rather than "fighting" to find a suture, it is best to position it in an easy access zone; like in football, we have to bring the ball back. When a suture is

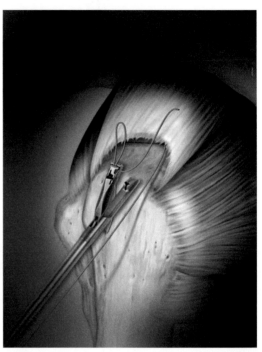

Fig. 5.35

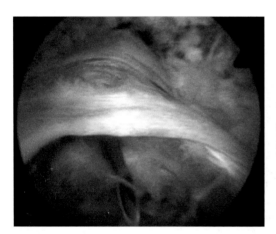

Fig. 5.33

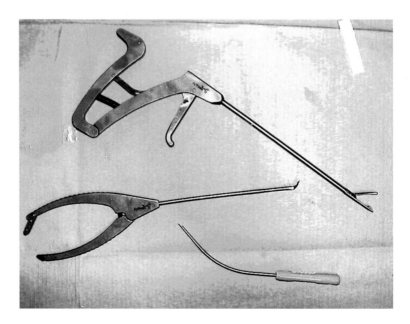

Fig. 5.34

passed, it must be placed into a waiting area where it is clearly visible (called the garage or waiting room). The easiest way is to use the surgical approach we used for placing the implants (Figs. 5.41, 5.42, and 5.43).

The sutures are waiting in an easily visible area.

In the case of delaminated cuff with two layers, we can reduce the lower sheet with the wire catch and pass with the needle at the same time. This is the "knife and fork" technique. This is not possible with a forceps for suturing the cuff.

For a small tear in a young patient, the double row is indicated.

For a proper tissue clamping, an analogy must be made with the closure of the skin. We correctly load the tissue by being perpendicular. This is a reason not to hesitate to vary surgical approaches. In this sense, the upper approach of Neviaser for damage to the supraspinatus is logical. The use of a simple curved needle is in line with this.

The second row is made with lateral sutures using impacted implants, which limits the number of sutures involved.

For small tears in young patients, we have evolved toward a technique that combines a median screwed implant with a suture and a lateral braided band forming a cerclage. The median suture ensures a compression on the first implant (Figs. 5.45, 5.46, 5.47, 5.48, and 5.49).

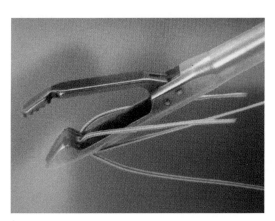

Fig. 5.36

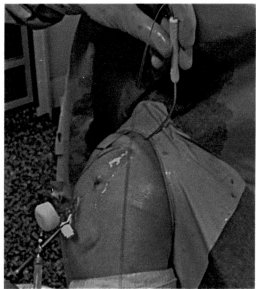

Fig. 5.38

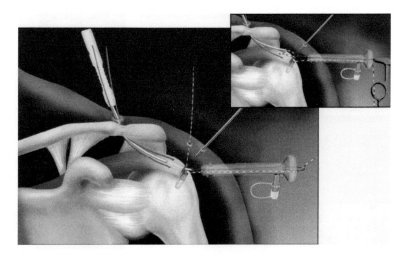

Fig. 5.37

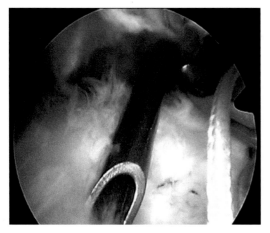

Fig. 5.39

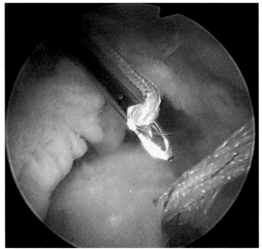

Fig. 5.42

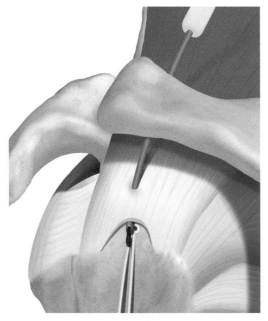

Fig. 5.40

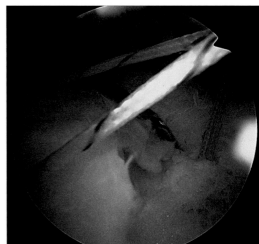

Fig. 5.43

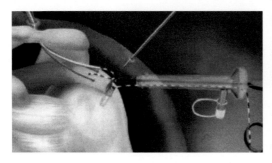

Fig. 5.41

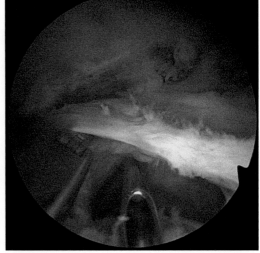

Fig. 5.44

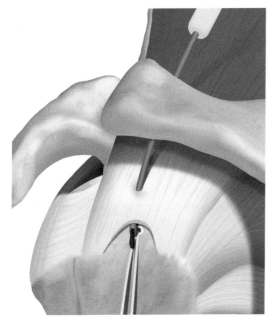

Fig. 5.45

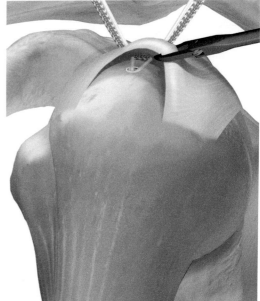

Fig. 5.47

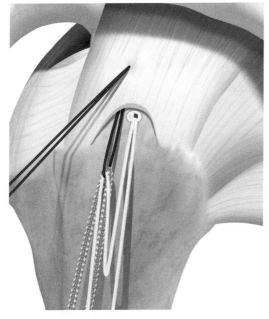

Fig. 5.46

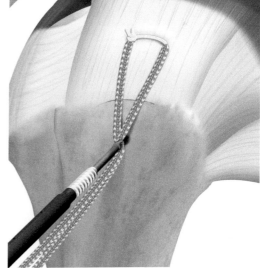

Fig. 5.48

This technique allows a double row to be made by only performing two passages through the cuff (it's the row and a half). Using a relay cable allows the suture and the "tape" to be passed simultaneously and without difficulty. Do not try to pass them in the needle, as they will block.

Here is how it actually appears; it is fast and effective because the initial decision to use the Banana allows a skillful tissue clamping. This technique is visible in the subscapularis video (Figs. 5.50, 5.51, 5.52, 5.53, and 5.54).

A tape can also be passed alone like a strapping, and this is the "SpeedFix" technique. But in this case, the absence of compression of the first row on the tuberosity creates a risk of unealing (Fig. 5.55).

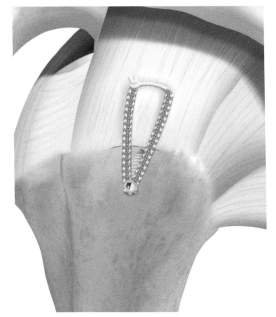

Fig. 5.49

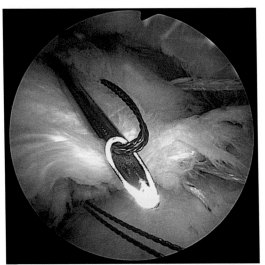

Fig. 5.51

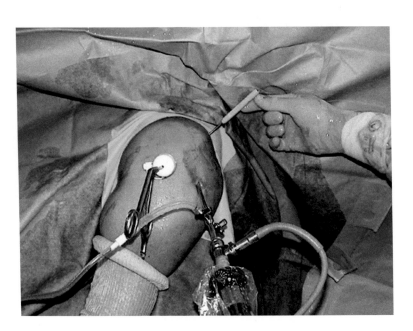

Fig. 5.50

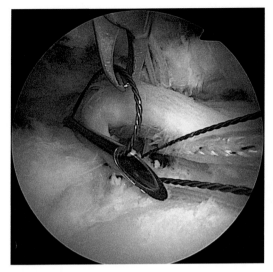

Fig. 5.52

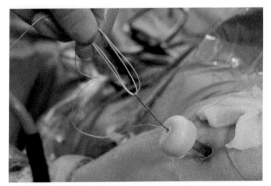

Fig. 5.53

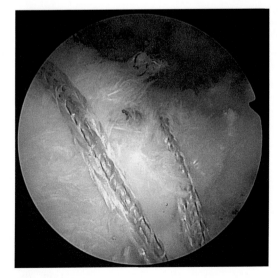

Fig. 5.54

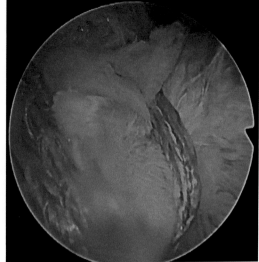

Fig. 5.55

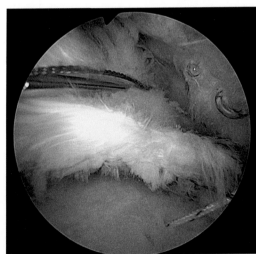

Fig. 5.56

For small- or medium-sized L-shaped tears, the simplified double-row technique can be used. But the orientation of the implants and the choice of work approach will depend on the initial analysis. Here is an example of L-shape at anterior corner. After surgery, a simple small point allows full closure of the vertical leg of the L-shape (Figs. 5.56, 5.57, 5.58, 5.59, 5.60, and 5.61).

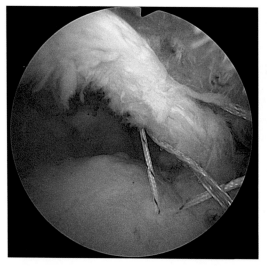

Fig. 5.57

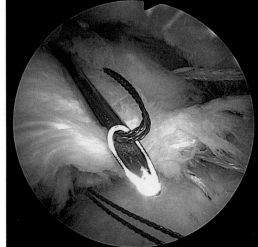

Fig. 5.59

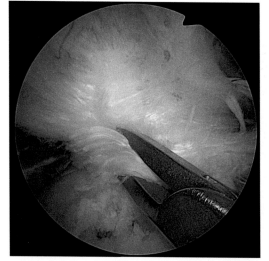

Fig. 5.58

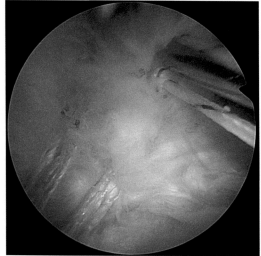

Fig. 5.60

For intermediate tears, the bridge technique is excellent. It can be carried out using wire or tape.

The tape has the advantage of reducing the shear effect, but its handling is more difficult and requires dedicated instrumentation (Figs. 5.62, 5.63, 5.64, 5.65, 5.66, and 5.67).

For these "bridges," the leg of the bridge must not be too broad, as an ear can be caught when tightening it. The technical principles remain the same; a good tissue compression of the insertion

or "footprint" zone, as can be seen in the final appearance (Figs. 5.68, 5.69, 5.70, 5.71, 5.72, 5.73, and 5.74).

Similarly, these "bridges" can be made with fiber tape; the principles are also the same as on this very delaminated cuff. You must be careful with the tension and pull lightly until the eye of the implant is buried. Laterally, we can use implants with titanium endpiece which avoids the tedious search for a small tunnel in a very lateral area. For this impaction, the

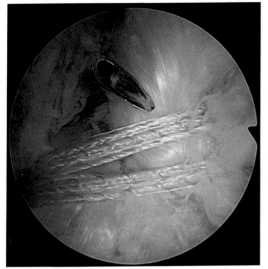

Fig. 5.61

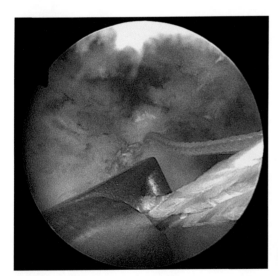

Fig. 5.62

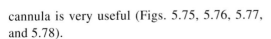

Fig. 5.63

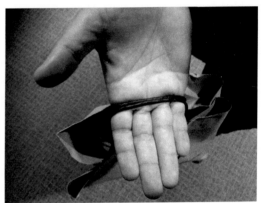

Fig. 5.64

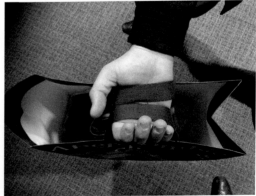

Fig. 5.65

cannula is very useful (Figs. 5.75, 5.76, 5.77, and 5.78).

For large tears, do not be alarmed by radiologists' reports. The sagittal view is sometimes reassuring, the "side to side" or "margin convergence" suture may be possible (Figs. 5.79, 5.80, 5.81, and 5.82).

For this patient, the frontal view is worrying, but the sagittal view (from proximal to distal) confirms what we see on the arthroscopic view that it is a large V-shaped tear!

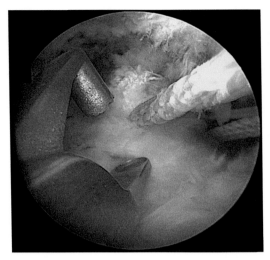

Fig. 5.66

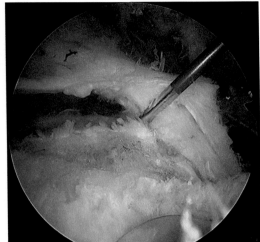

Fig. 5.69

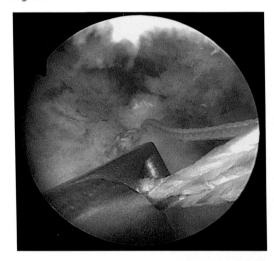

Fig. 5.67

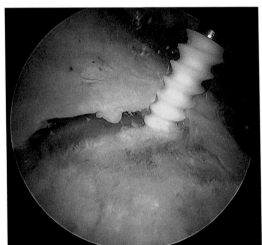

Fig. 5.70

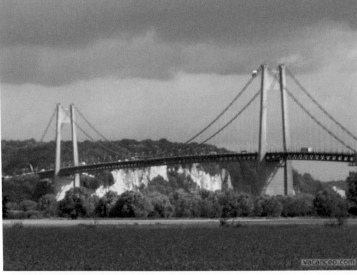

Fig. 5.68

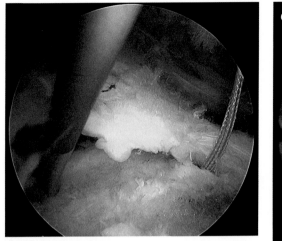

Fig. 5.71

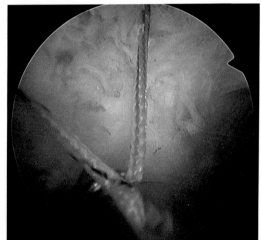

Fig. 5.72   (continued)

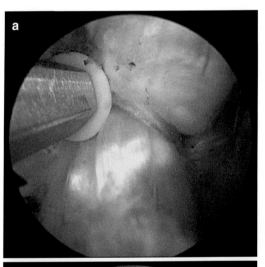

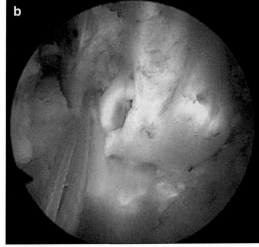

Fig. 5.72

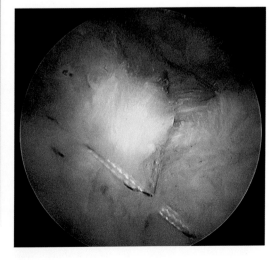

Fig. 5.73

Fig. 5.74

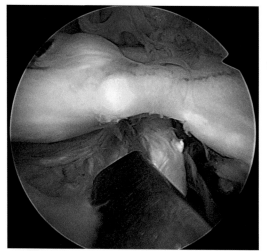

Fig. 5.75

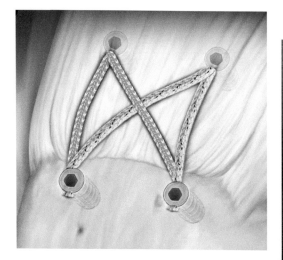

Fig. 5.76

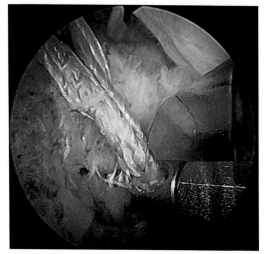

Fig. 5.77

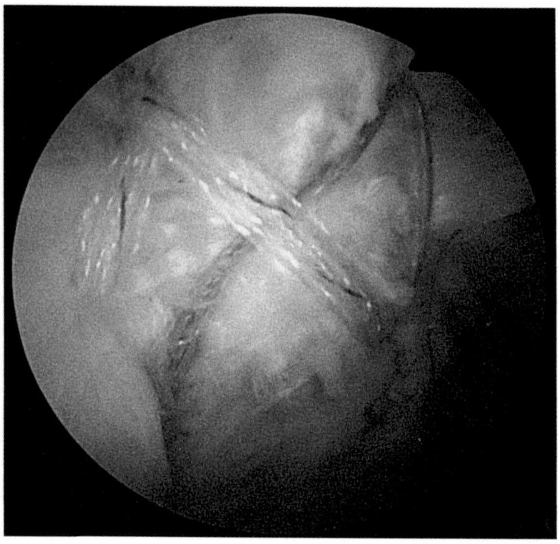

Fig. 5.78

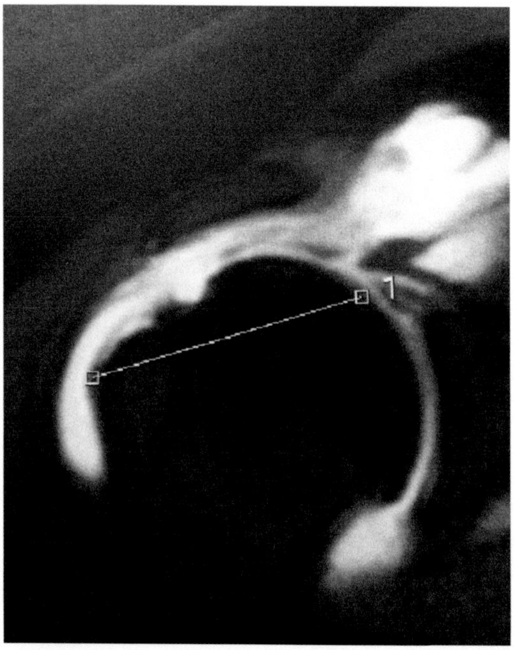

Fig. 5.79

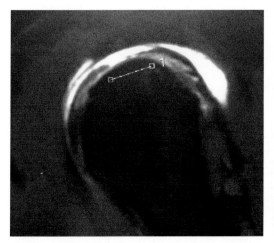

Fig. 5.80

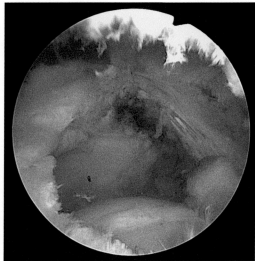

Fig. 5.82

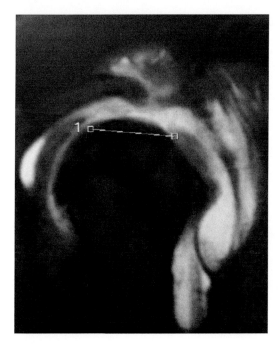

Fig. 5.81

In this case, we must maintain the principle of proper tissue clamping. The best way, as with a needle holder, is to be perpendicular to the bank. As well as the Neviaser approach, you must use a posterior approach: either the former optical approach or an approach more inward if the tear is very retracted. For the anterior layer, use a forward approach of the clavicle by going along it

and staying outside the coracoid to be in the safe zone. Before using the three portals and beginning on this type of patient, mock training is recommended. The needle will seem tangential and yet it will be perpendicular to the banks of the tear (Figs. 5.83, 5.84, 5.85, 5.86, and 5.87).

Side to side sutures, in theory (Figs. 5.88, 5.89, 5.90, and 5.91)

In practice, this "side to side" or "margin convergence" technique limits tedious dissections and reduces tension and possibly the risk of secondary necrosis. This type of suture is not perfectly anatomical, but its results on pain and function are surprising (Figs. 5.92, 5.93, 5.94, and 5.95).

With the first "side to side" points made, we are astonished by the reduction of this large tear. We are then "brought" to an intermediate size tear closed here on a double row (Figs. 5.96 and 5.97).

Another technique is lacing it in the manner of a sports shoe or corset. We transfile a fiber tape into the tear and we produce the tension at each passage. The final appearance is amazing; you must alternately reverse the direction of the relay cable, so that you can always pass the tissue according to the needle holder principle (Figs. 5.98, 5.99, 5.100, and 5.101).

Fig. 5.83

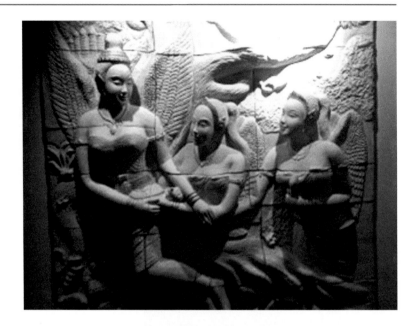

Fig. 5.84

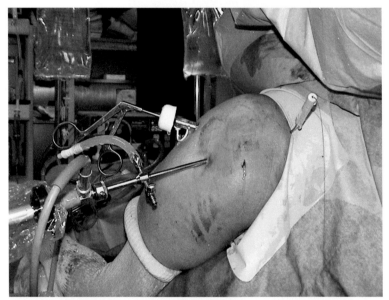

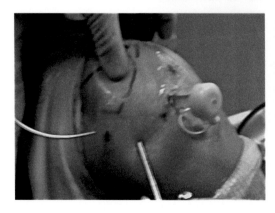

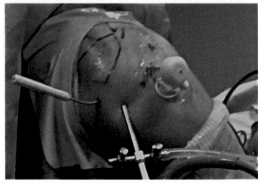

Fig. 5.86

Fig. 5.85

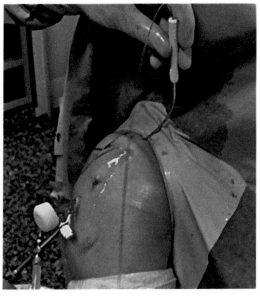

Fig. 5.87

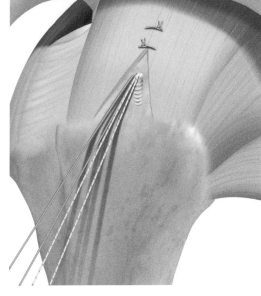

Fig. 5.89

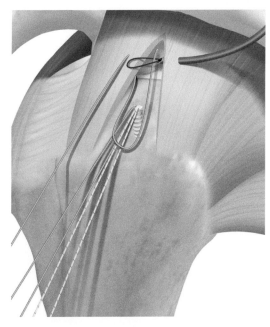

Fig. 5.88

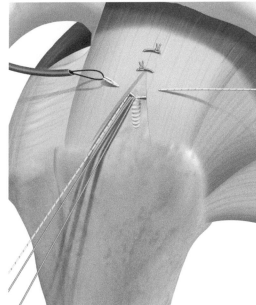

Fig. 5.90

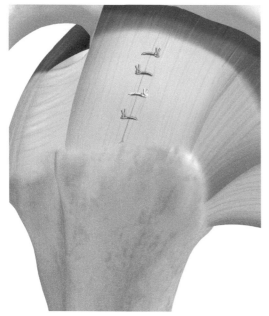

Fig. 5.91

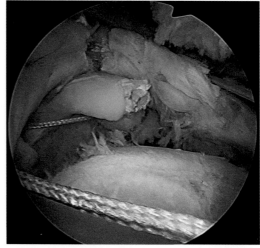

Fig. 5.93

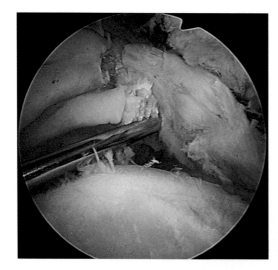

Fig. 5.92

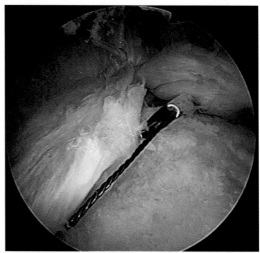

Fig. 5.94

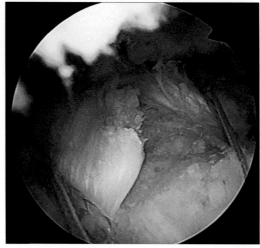

Fig. 5.95

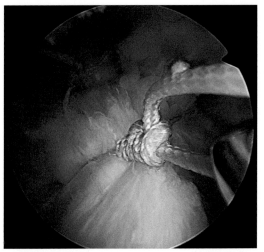

Fig. 5.96

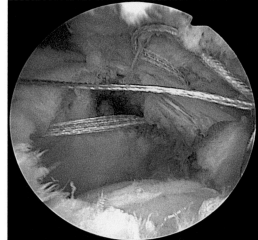

Fig. 5.99

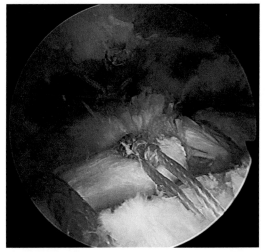

Fig. 5.97

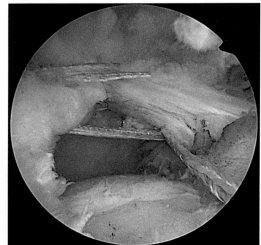

Fig. 5.100

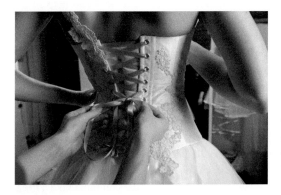

Fig. 5.98

Sometimes the cuff is impossible to re-close, the tenotomy will have an analgesic role, and depending on age, a flap will possibly be offered under arthroscopy. Whatever the cost, it is pointless to re-close poor quality tissue. When you look back and you see the teres minor, it often means game over (Fig. 5.102).

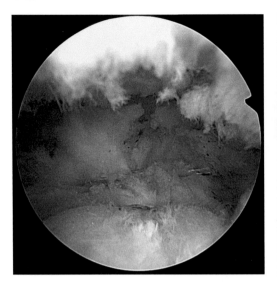

Fig. 5.101

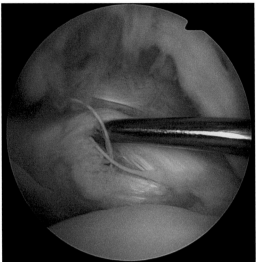

Fig. 5.103

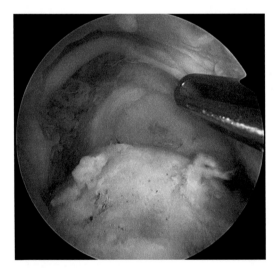

Fig. 5.102

5.3   The Subscapularis

Repairing subscapularis lesions still has a difficult reputation. It is probably due to this that we
tend not to see them. However, if we remain true
to our principles of simplicity, these lesions can
ultimately prove easier to repair than we had
thought. As we gain in confidence, we start to
detect them with rigor. And finally when that
becomes a necessity, it will be a real pleasure to
tackle them.

Here are some lesions called "hidden."
Sometimes we have to go through the bicipital
groove to detect them. We can also sensitize the
examination by playing on the shoulder's rotation, and the RI allows an improved visualization
of the lesion as the shoulder is relaxed.

It is not enough to look; you must palpate. In
Fig. 5.19, we visualize the "comma sign." The
comma is actually the coracohumeral ligament or
rather the anterior extension of the supraspinatus.
This latter migrates inward and makes this
comma that you must respect in the repair (Figs.
5.103, 5.104, 5.105, and 5.106).

Once the lesion is diagnosed, it suffices to
apply our basic principles.

Choose the surgical approach that will allow
the repair. This can be done with the help of an
OL needle; an anterolateral approach is that
which is most often used. Leaving the scope by
posterior approach is most of the time well
adapted for lesions 2/3 greater. In addition, a lateral approach for the scope will be more suitable,
but it is rarely necessary (Figs. 5.107 and 5.108).

The scope is left by posterior approach, an
upper approach of reduction (traction clamp),
anterolateral approach for the cannula, and anterior approach for the wire pass.

As for the supraspinatus, you must take a little
time to perform the anterior bursectomy and the

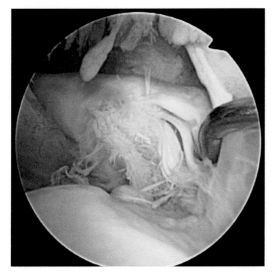

Fig. 5.104

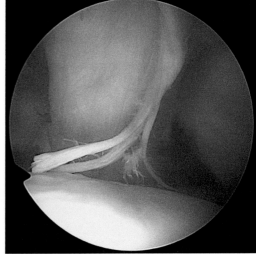

Fig. 5.106

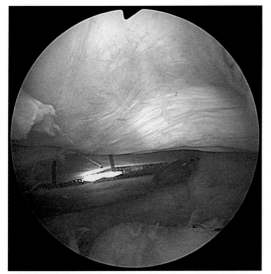

Fig. 5.105

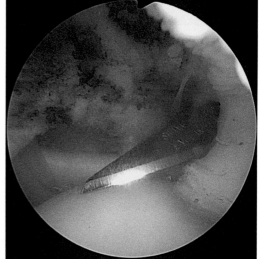

Fig. 5.107

dissection that will allow the subscapularis to be mobilized.

As with any action on the cuff, this time it is important to quickly find your sutures (Fig. 5.109).

To make a double row, we use the same technique as for the supraspinatus (Fig. 5.110).

To facilitate the repair of the subscapularis, a tenodesis of the tendon along the biceps under the bicipital groove is recommended; this will be detailed in a later chapter. Due to the significant forces present, it may be preferable to repair on a double row. The technique we use is simplified because lateral access is sometimes difficult. The use of knotless fixation implants is interesting in this respect.

To properly access the inner section of the insertion zone, we put the RE, and we maintain this position for placing the first row of implants. Here everything is done through the anterolateral cannula (Figs. 5.111 and 5.112).

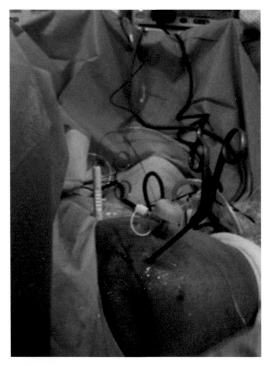

Fig. 5.108

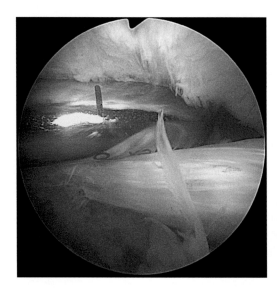

Fig. 5.109

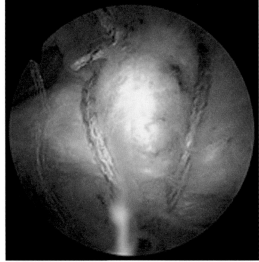

Fig. 5.110

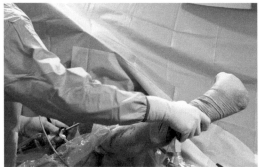

Fig. 5.111

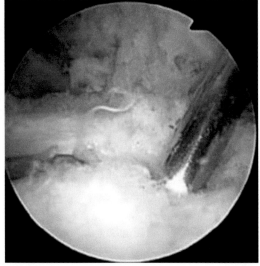

Fig. 5.112

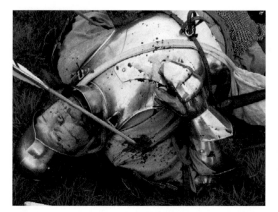

Fig. 5.113

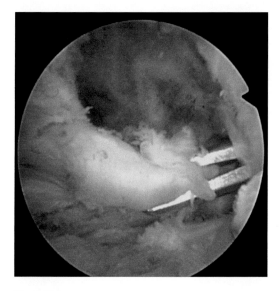

Fig. 5.114

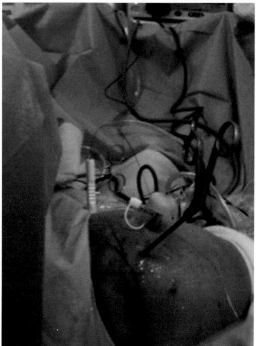

Fig. 5.115

an arrow), and we target the posterior scope by looking at our hands (Figs. 5.113, 5.114, and 5.115).

Once the tendon is transfixed, we can pass the relay cable, and the pulling clamp allows us to recuperate it inside the cannula.

As for the repair of the simplified double row, we pass the suture of the screwed implant and a braided tape (Fiber Tape®) simultaneously.

The wires are left in front (in the service station or the waiting room). They are recuperated inside the cannula. It is important to have performed a good cleaning of this anterior area to easily find the sutures again (Figs. 5.116 and 5.117).

The reduction is performed in neutral rotation; we begin by the lateral stay on the tape according to the SpeedFix® technique (Figs. 5.118 and 5.119).

In Fig. 5.119, we notice the wires of the medial row "waiting." Compression on the first row is then carried out by conventional knot. We can then see the final appearance of this suture (Figs. 5.120 and 5.121).

With the shoulder in external rotation and having freshened the greater tuberosity of the humerus, it is easy to put the first row (screwed implants).

In order to clamp a sufficient amount of tissue, the prehensile clamp allows the tendon of the subscapularis to be put under lateral traction. Indeed, in this case, it would be dangerous to come from "inside."

Then, once the tracted tendon is outside, we can transfix it with the help of the Banana Lasso. It is understood that the release stage is important, but this must be performed without devascularization.

This approach is a bit unusual of course just outside the coracoid process. We are sagittal (like

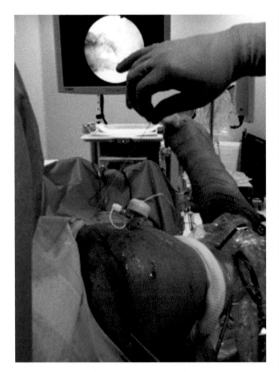

Fig. 5.116

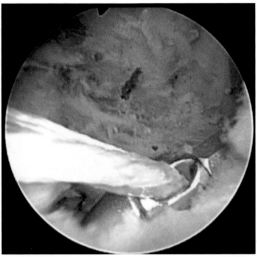

Fig. 5.118

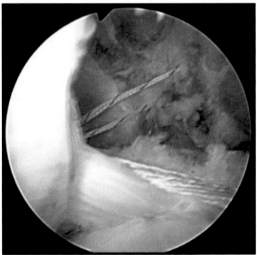

Fig. 5.119

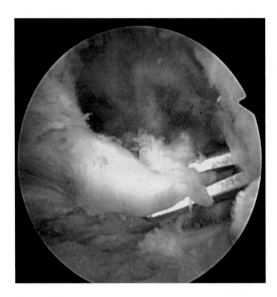

Fig. 5.117

Through a lateral approach for the scope, we see the final appearance. On the inspection radiography, we clearly see the lateral implant and the tunnel under the groove corresponding to the tenodesis (Figs. 5.122, 5.123, and 5.124).

For small tears, a simple cerclage on a simple lateral row can be achieved. And for those who have had the patience to read this far, here's a little "trick" to avoid losing your sutures; just fold them at the end! (Figs. 5.125 and 5.126)

This tendon, which is the one most often broken by trauma, provides good healing at a minimally esthetic price (Fig. 5.127).

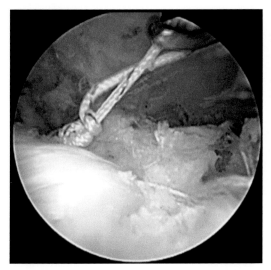

Fig. 5.120

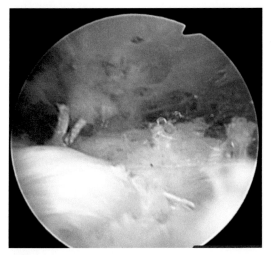

Fig. 5.121

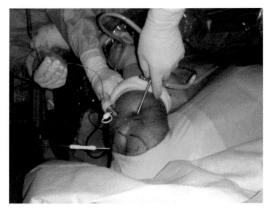

Fig. 5.122

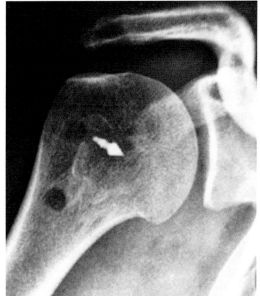

Fig. 5.123

Fig. 5.124

5.4   The Biceps

To dare is sometimes to be able to.

The tendon of the long biceps is one of the actors of the rotator cuff, but it also has its own pathology.

In the case of pathology of the cuff, the tendon of the long biceps must always be evaluated. Clinically the O'Brien maneuver as well as the

Fig. 5.125

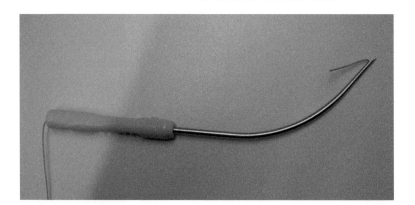

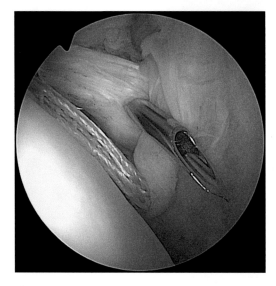

Fig. 5.126

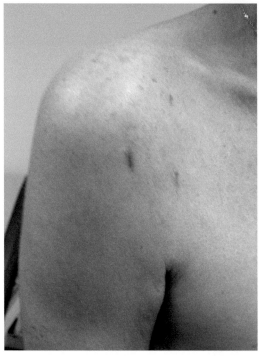

Fig. 5.127

imaging review arouse interest before the surgery; we must seek a subluxation, a laminated or thickened appearance; dynamic ultrasound no doubt has its place in this review.

Here are some examples of biceps that attract attention before the surgery (Figs. 5.128, 5.129, and 5.130).

Once inside the shoulder, certain pathologies are evident such as here (Figs. 5.131 and 5.132).

But **beware**, sometimes the diagnosis is more difficult and dynamic palpation is required, as in the case of inflammatory biceps or SLAP detected with the help of the probe (Figs. 5.133 and 5.134).

The hourglass biceps is sometimes a hidden lesion, and you are surprised when the lesion is externalized. In fact, during the arthroscopy, the

"misleading" biceps presents itself under its good profile! Dynamic exploration in anterior elevation that seeks a blockage at the entrance of the groove once again provides an important diagnostic element (Figs. 5.135 and 5.136).

There are then two possibilities for this biceps: a simple tenotomy or a tenodesis.

Tenotomy is simple so popular, but in some cases, it can lead to the famous "Popeye sign." There are no esthetic drawbacks; the cramps and pains are not easy to treat (botulinum toxin injec-

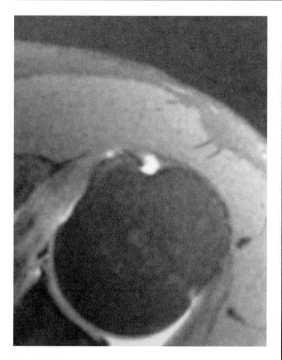

Fig. 5.128

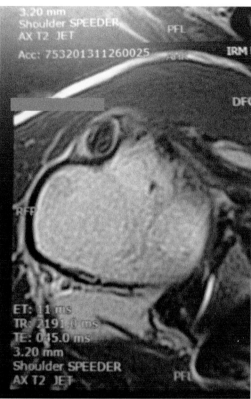

Fig. 5.129

tion). Sometimes with the simple tenotomy (even if it is self-locking), the patient still has pain during the O'Brien maneuver. These pains are probably due to a residual inflammation of the biceps but also to receptors present in the groove (Figs. 5.137 and 5.138).

This is why we have turned toward a tenodesis under the bicipital groove. It is not systematically performed, but it is indicated for active and slender patients. Finally, do not limit this technique, as it is also very useful for repairing damage to the subscapularis. Without biceps in the groove, the subscapularis will be repaired more easily and efficiently.

For this technique, it is important to situate the groove during palpation. We tend to situate it too inward. Dynamic palpation in rotation allows us to locate it. The surgical approaches are also drawn from both sides, lateral for the scope and medial for the instrumentation, at two subacromial fingerbreadths (Figs. 5.139 and 5.140).

The first stage of this technique is intra-articular, and it consists of securing the biceps with a single needle (there are no acrobatics to be performed for passing a wire). The tenotomy is then carried out (Figs. 5.141 and 5.142).

We then apply the same principles that we have seen repeatedly. We must create the space under the deltoid. To do this, we will put the arm in anterior elevation; while looking at our hands we "touch" the end of the mandrel and the shaver and the humerus before putting the scope. This is time saved! We are not required to have three screens for performing this technique, but ergonomic installation with a screen opposite is always pleasant (Figs. 5.143 and 5.144).

Then we need a bit of patience to find the bicipital groove. Due to the glenohumeral stage, it bulges most of the time. The use of the shaver and the thermal probe is recommended; this area is in fact well vascularized. The transverse fibers of the groove are an excellent reference. We can then open it up to visualize the tendon (Figs. 5.145, 5.146, 5.147, 5.148, and 5.149).

Fig. 5.130

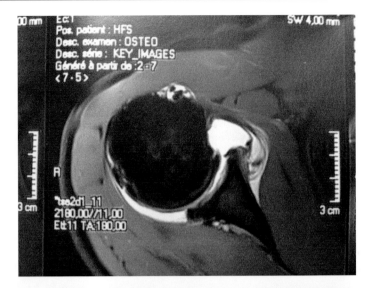

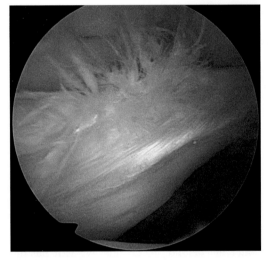

Fig. 5.131

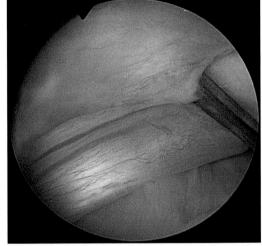

Fig. 5.133

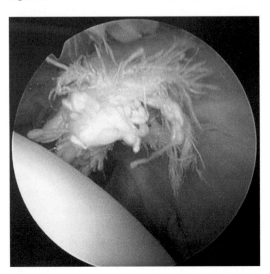

Fig. 5.132

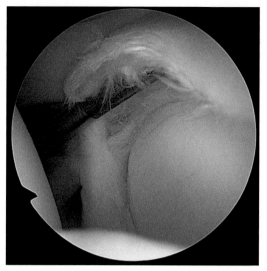

Fig. 5.134

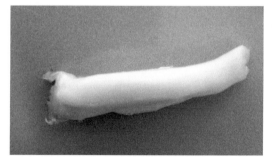

Fig. 5.135

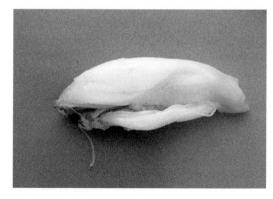

Fig. 5.136

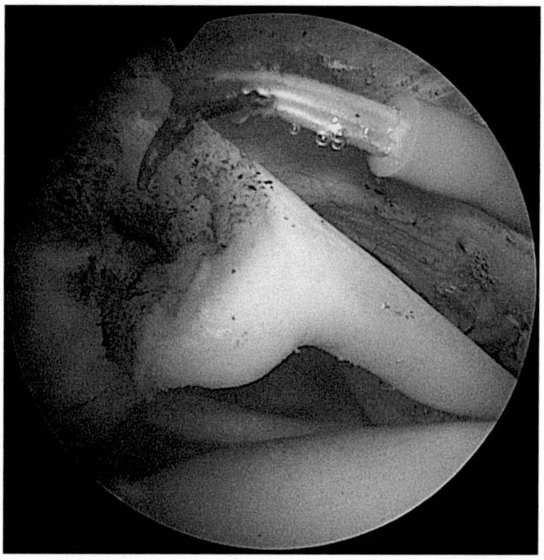

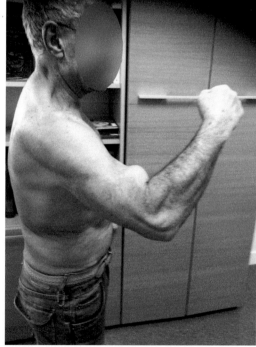

Fig. 5.137

Fig. 5.138

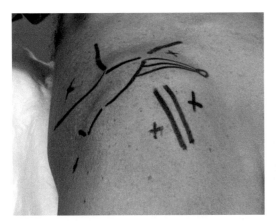

Fig. 5.139

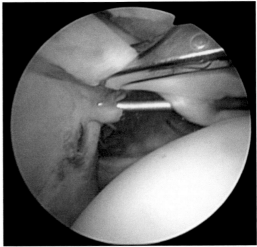

Fig. 5.141

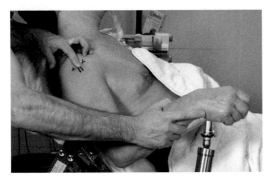

Fig. 5.140

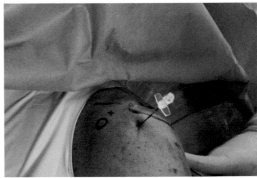

Fig. 5.142

With the clamper, we must then externalize the tendon and secure the Kocher so not to lose it. The threading is done after a section of 3 cm which means the tension of the biceps can be maintained thus avoiding excessive tension, which is a source of pain or stiffness of the elbow. We must then simply calibrate it to decide on the size of the tunnel (Figs. 5.150, 5.151, 5.152, 5.153, and 5.154).

To make the tunnel under the groove, we have a simple instrumentation, without viewfinder or engine. We make the 20 cm blind tunnel using the tarot after simple marking by the needle (Figs. 5.155, 5.156, 5.157, 5.158, and 5.159).

Using the "sweeve lock®" (usually 6.25), the tendon is pushed into socket; then all there is to do is to fix it by screwing. **Be careful not to over-tighten** as the best attachment is on the cortical bone. For the same reason, it is important to clean the entrance of the tunnel rather than enlarge it. We will use resorbable screws with or without hydroxylapatite according to our beliefs (Figs. 5.160, 5.161, 5.162, 5.163, 5.164, 5.165, 5.166, 5.167, and 5.168).

If the biceps tendon is thin, we can double it up by threading in that way. In this case, we will not cut its end to avoid excessive tension (Fig. 5.169).

Here is the scar appearance at a distance, the radio inspection, and MRI of the patient (Figs. 5.170, 5.171, and 5.172).

If the bone is of unexpectedly poor quality, we can use a larger diameter screw or double the tendon in the tunnel by passing a suture around upstream from the threading.

This technique is simple, elegant, and reliable provided we follow our rules: **look carefully, take your time, follow the steps, and don't forget to breathe!**

Fig. 5.143

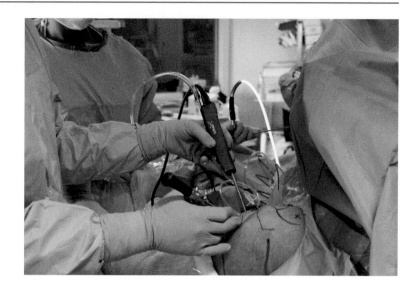

Fig. 5.144

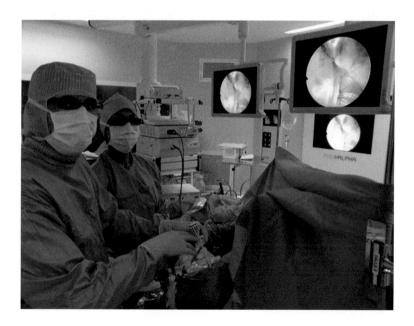

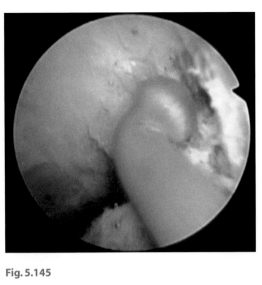

Fig. 5.145

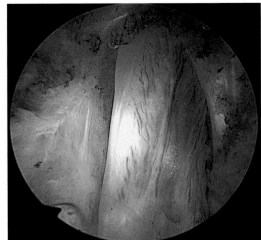

Fig. 5.148

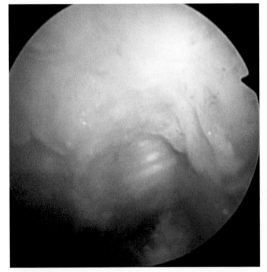

Fig. 5.146

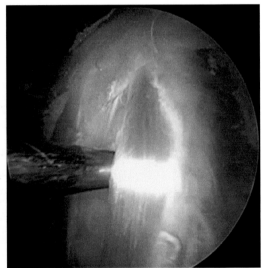

Fig. 5.149

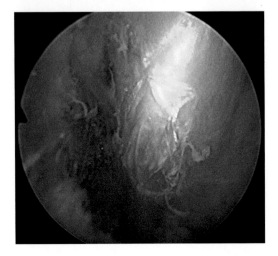

Fig. 5.147

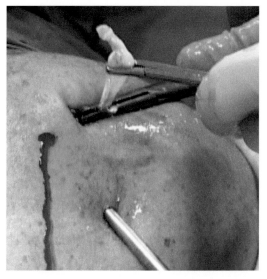

Fig. 5.150

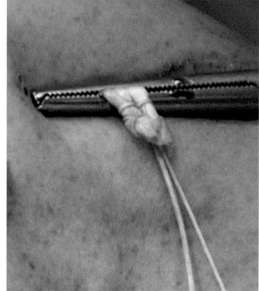

Fig. 5.152

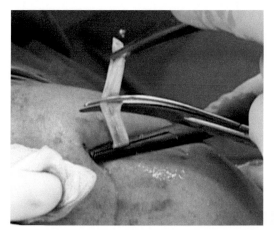

Fig. 5.151

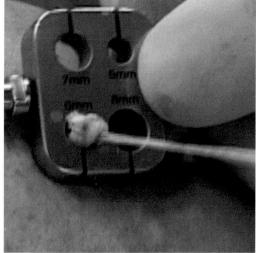

Fig. 5.153

5.5   Instability and the Arthroscopic Bankart

The unstable shoulder is a condition that **most often affects athletes or very active people**. This is why it is very difficult to promise a forgotten shoulder.

As in all the techniques we have discussed, we must be rigorous. But we must know how to select patients and not put ourselves at risk by being too audacious in our indications, even if you become more confident. The ISIS rating is a very good guard. Caution is the order of the day!

To select the **lucky winners of arthroscopy**, avoid patients who are too young, doing sports in competition, and with heavy demands on the shoulder. Hyperlaxity will also be eliminated by a simple search of an external hyper-rotation (> at 95°). Obviously a bone defect of the glenoid or an engaging notch will also be a contraindication.

In these selected patients, it is necessary to present the advantages of the arthroscopy, which are a more anatomical shoulder and above all the absence of subscapularis aggression. But you must not hide the risk of recurrence from them which, despite this selection, remains more significant than for open-cast techniques.

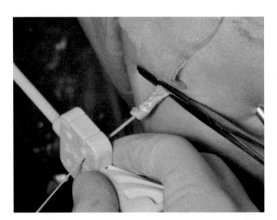

Fig. 5.154

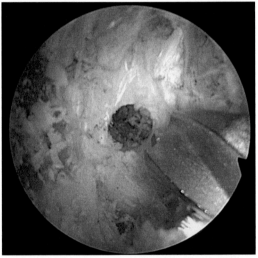

Fig. 5.156

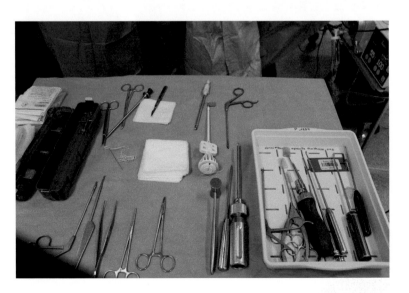

Fig. 5.155

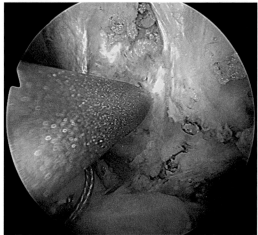

Fig. 5.157

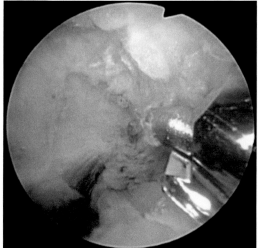

Fig. 5.158

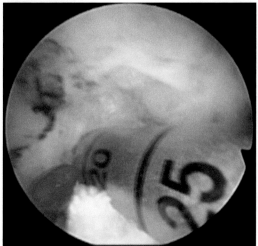

Fig. 5.159

Fig. 5.160

Fig. 5.161

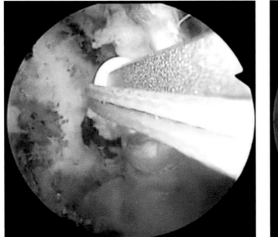

Fig. 5.162

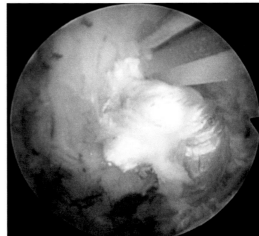

Fig. 5.163

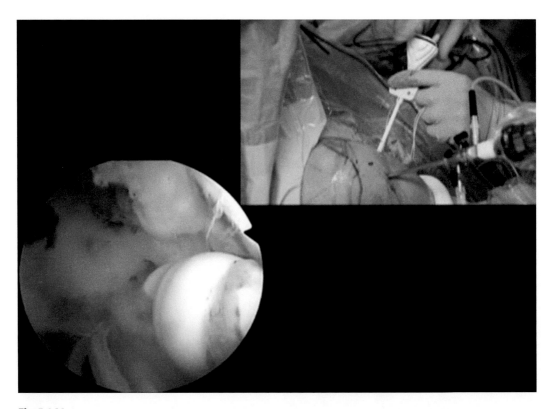

Fig. 5.164

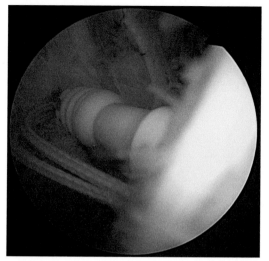

Fig. 5.165

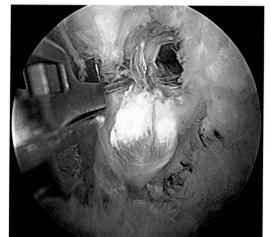

Fig. 5.166

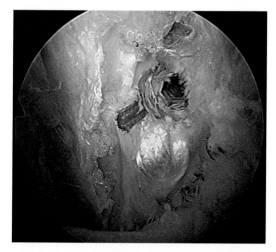

Fig. 5.167

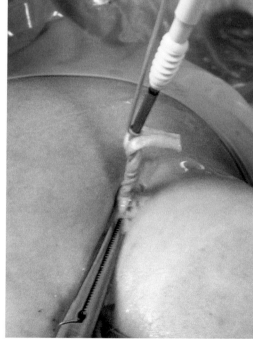

Fig. 5.168

Fig. 5.169

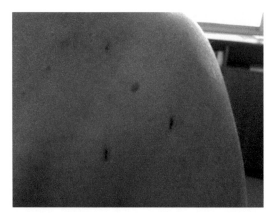

Fig. 5.170

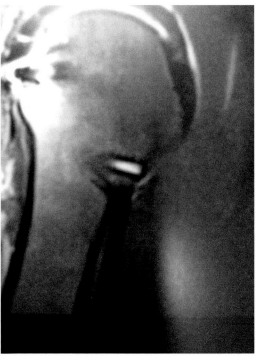

Fig. 5.172

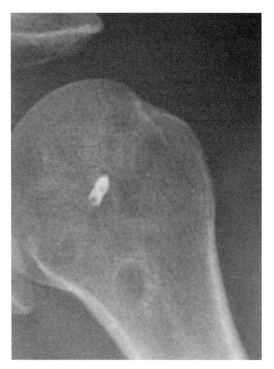

Fig. 5.171

For these patients, we need to give ourselves the best possible chances of success. A good surgical technique begins with a rigorous installation.

To maximize the exposure of the LGHI, lateral recumbency with traction device, but particularly decoaptation, is more suitable (Figs. 5.173, 5.174, and 5.175).

The posterior approach, for the scope, will be willingly lateraled, so the scope by a leverage

effect on the humeral head allows you a better workspace (Figs. 5.176, 5.177, and 5.178).

For the anterior approach, by taking your time, you can perform it from outside in with the needle. The incidence must be properly oblique to facilitate work on the labrum but also the positioning of the implants. The needle should "mimic" the surgery to be certain that the surgical approach will be satisfactory. Once enabled, you can position one or more cannulas (Figs. 5.179, 5.180, and 5.181).

Then comes the time for exploration. **We must be careful because sometimes we may discover a contraindication for this technique.**

We search a notch which must remain nonbinding, a labral lesion on the humeral side (HAGL) which must remain small sized and a damage to the glenoid which is sometimes a cartilage damage (GLAD). This damage should be noted in the operating report (Figs. 5.182, 5.183, and 5.184).

The work can then begin. **The steps are well known, but you must take your time.** A Bankart too quickly done ensures a recurrence!

Fig. 5.173

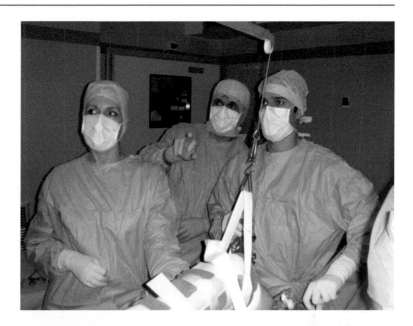

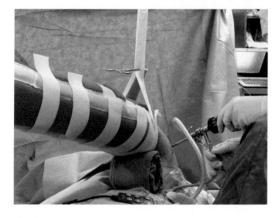

Fig. 5.174

The first stage is the analysis of the lesion to be repaired; a superoexternal approach is recommended (Figs. 5.185, 5.186, 5.187, and 5.188).

The second stage is a dissection that consists of aggravating the lesion. For this, we use the cutting elevator; it can be used with a mallet, because then we detach small bony pellets that will facilitate healing. This dissection should be carried out until the muscle fibers of the subscapularis are visualized. At the end of this stage, when we turn off the water, the labrum should reduce all by itself (Figs. 5.189, 5.190, and 5.191).

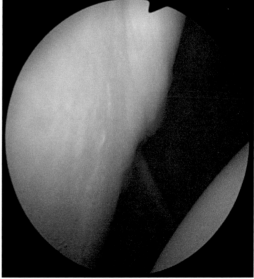

Fig. 5.175

It is then necessary to prepare the bone curette or the bone awl to facilitate healing (Fig. 5.192).

The next stage is the passage of the sutures. We must keep in mind the goal of reducing the labrum but also of a plasty of the capsule which does not limit the external rotation. In fact, it is necessary that this plasty is vertically upward. The passage from the lowest point is very important in this respect.

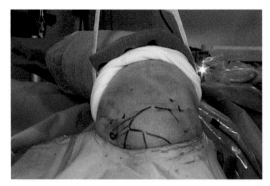

Fig. 5.176

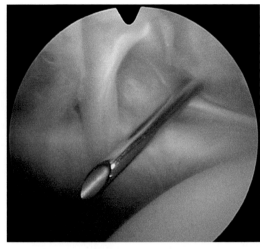

Fig. 5.179

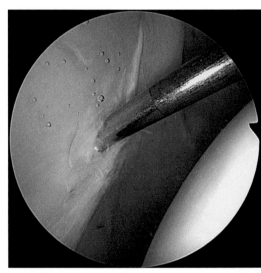

Fig. 5.180

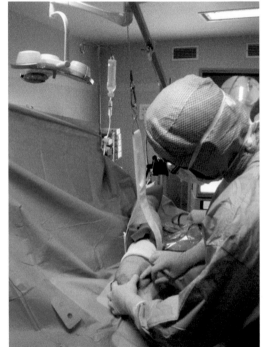

Fig. 5.177

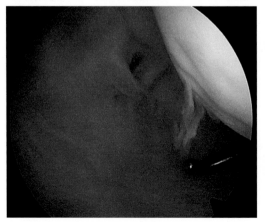

Fig. 5.178

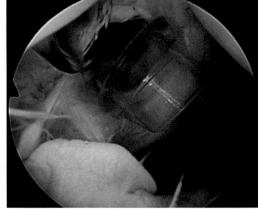

Fig. 5.181

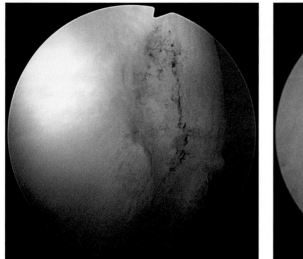

Fig. 5.182

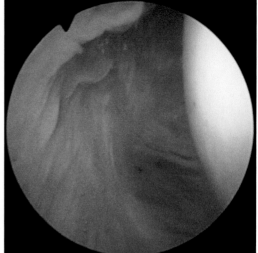

Fig. 5.184

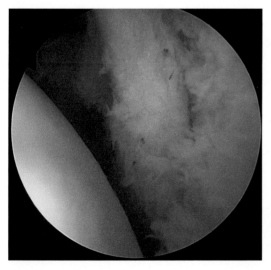

Fig. 5.183

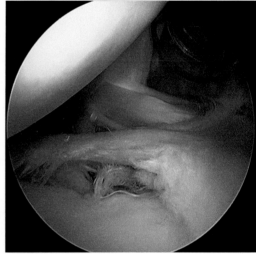

Fig. 5.185

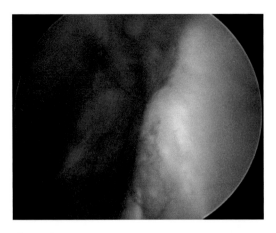

Fig. 5.186

For this passage, you must not hesitate to use a temporary manual decoaptation. A traction point passed through the upper cannula also allows a better grip.

We can use a posterolateral approach for the wire pass. Be careful to follow the rules when performing this approach; there are risks of damage to the circumflex if this approach is done without caution (Figs. 5.193, 5.194, 5.195, and 5.196).

To do the plasty, all you have to do is take two sutures during the first passage. The second suture passage is therefore performed 8–10 mm above. The implant was positioned at "5 hours,"

Fig. 5.187

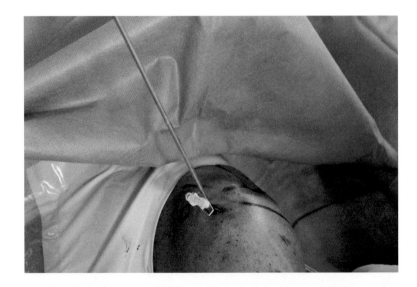

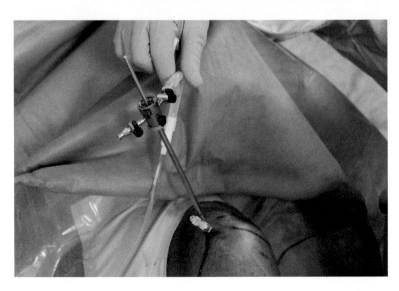

Fig. 5.188

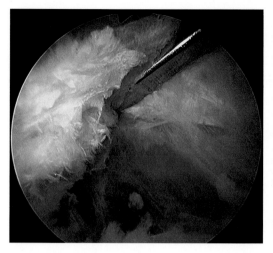

Fig. 5.189

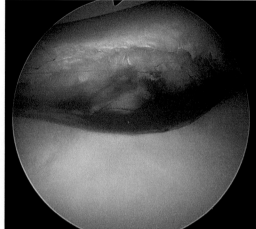

Fig. 5.191

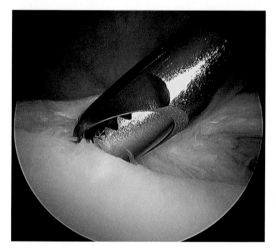

Fig. 5.190

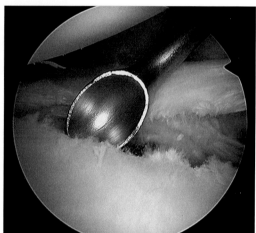

Fig. 5.192

slightly overlapping the cartilage. For this passage, we can use the anterior approach (Figs. 5.197, 5.198, and 5.199).

Here is the final appearance which we call "bumper." You have to position three implants on average. The upper implant improves the strength of the whole like the press stud on the anorak (Fig. 5.200).

In the case of cartilage lesion, we can perform it on the oblique tip of the micro-fractures and "mount" the labrum to be sutured onto the glenoid. We must also warn the patient of these lesions which can ultimately become a source of pain (Figs. 5.201 and 5.202).

Finally in the case of a notch, we can use filling which, after freshening, allows the infraspinatus to be attached to prevent engagement (Figs. 5.203, 5.204, and 5.205).

Fig. 5.193

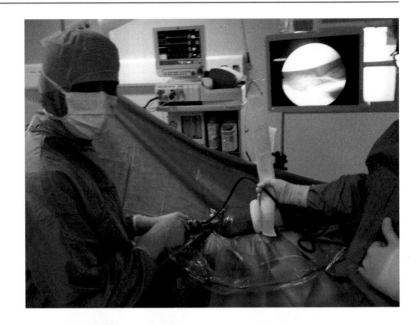

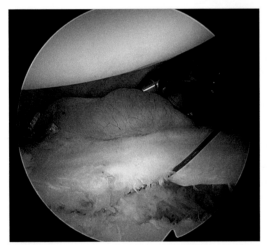

Fig. 5.194

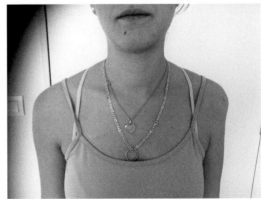

Fig. 5.196

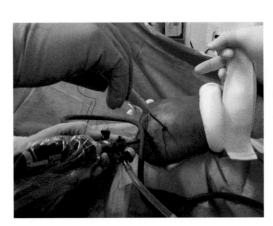

Fig. 5.195

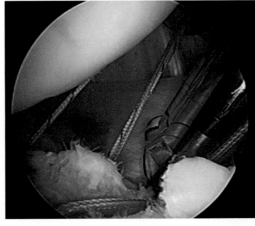

Fig. 5.197

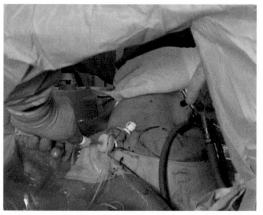

Fig. 5.198

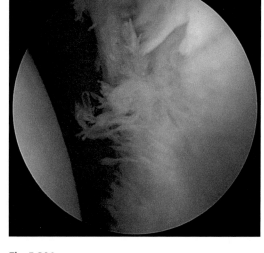

Fig. 5.201

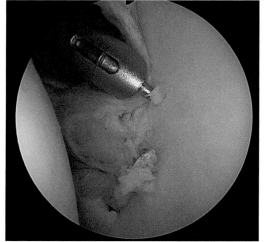

Fig. 5.199

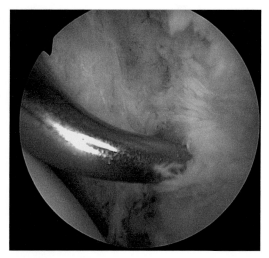

Fig. 5.202

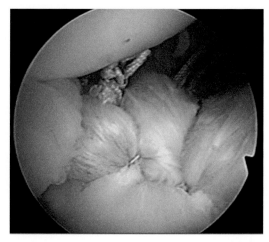

Fig. 5.200

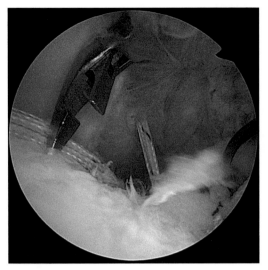

Fig. 5.203

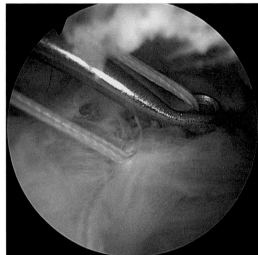

Fig. 5.205

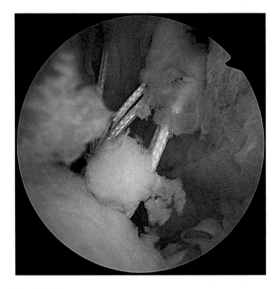

Fig. 5.204

Less Frequent Surgeries

6

6.1 The Acromioclavicular

We believe that the principles listed in the preceding chapters allow us to take a step back and will provide us with more tips to achieve successful surgeries.

Acromioclavicular osteoarthritis

When it is clinically and radiologically symptomatic, it sometimes requires the resection of the outer ¼ of the clavicle (Figs. 6.1 and 6.2).

Before starting these less frequent surgeries, it is recommended to perform a mock repetition (we will look at that for the release of the supra-scapular nerve) which allows you to reflect on surgical approaches.

For the resection of the outer ¼, we start like for an acromioplasty, but the visual display will be optimized by lateraling the approach for the strong oblique of the scope upward (Figs. 6.3 and 6.4).

An important tip for the above work approach is to perform it a good distance away at 3–4 cm under the clavicle. This avoids the risk of fistula.

The external optical approach allows a good visualization of the acromioclavicular joint (Figs. 6.5 and 6.6).

We can begin the resection with the round burr, which is the most appropriate. One of the "tricks" is to hold the clavicle with the thumb, which prevents it vibrating at the same time, which renders the resection tedious. After surgery, we can use our thumb to feel whether the resection is complete.

Fluoroscopic control by the anterior approach ensures that the resection is complete.

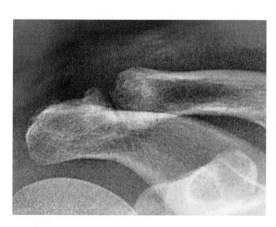

Fig. 6.1

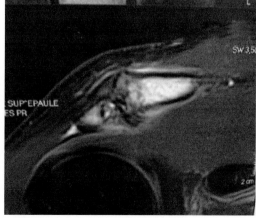

Fig. 6.2

O. Courage, *Shoulder Arthroscopy: How to Succeed!*, DOI 10.1007/978-3-319-23648-3_6

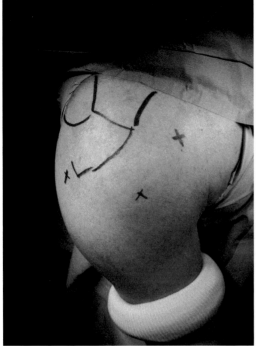

Fig. 6.3

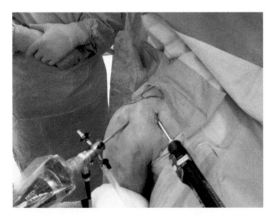

Fig. 6.4

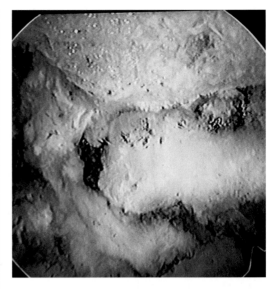

Fig. 6.5

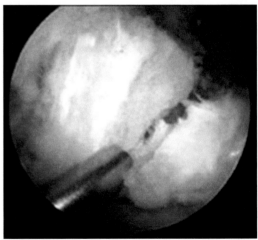

Fig. 6.6

Here is the radiological and esthetic result (Figs. 6.7 and 6.8).

Acromioclavicular instability

As for the resection, for the instability it is primordial that we respect our principles, choosing surgical approaches carefully and giving ourselves good exposure. The scope will be placed here by an anterolateral approach toward the coracoid process. The preparation of the coracoid is very important to avoid the unpleasant surprises of the "incomplete tunnel" (Figs. 6.9, 6.10, and 6.11).

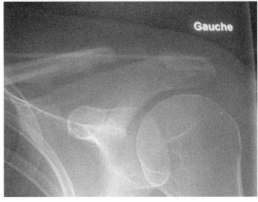

Fig. 6.7

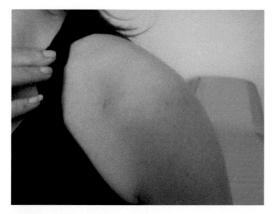

Fig. 6.8

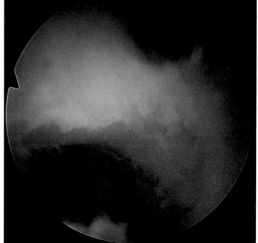

Fig. 6.11

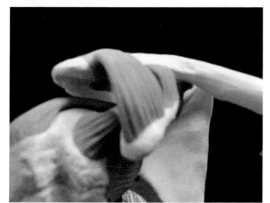

Fig. 6.9

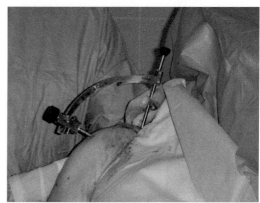

Fig. 6.12

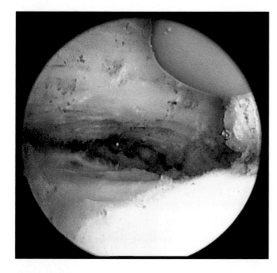

Fig. 6.10

As in ligament surgery, we must use the view-finders. The simpler and the more rigid they are, the more reliable they are. For that reason, this surgery is close to knee ligamentoplasties (Fig. 6.12).

The endobuttons must be inspected, as well as the tunnels. Here is a good example (Figs. 6.13, 6.14, and 6.15).

After surgery, we see the result with a ligament reinforcement at the gracilis in a chronic laxity (Figs. 6.16 and 6.17).

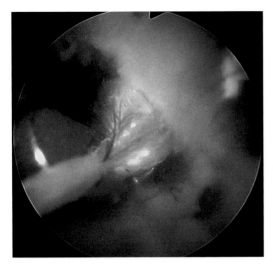

Fig. 6.13

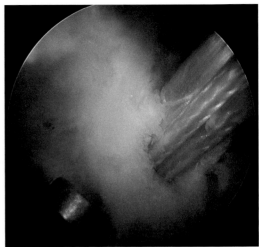

Fig. 6.15

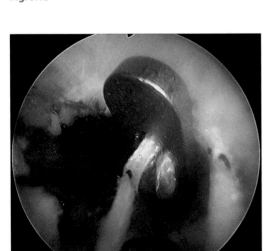

Fig. 6.14

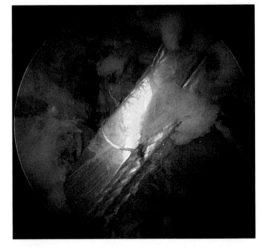

Fig. 6.16

6.2   The Subscapularis Nerve

The release of the suprascapular nerve

This operation can frighten, yet by respecting the right principles, you will be surprised to find yourself having performed it without incident. Repetition is essential here, as this surgery is seldom performed. Before operating this navigator, you had better be sure of your stroke (Figs. 6.18, 6.19, and 6.20).

By following on the model of the upper edge of the coracoid process, we find the recess and its transverse ligament (Figs. 6.21 and 6.22).

It is sufficient to section the transverse ligament by passing "en piquet" using the *Neviaser* approach and finally releasing the nerve (Figs. 6.23 and 6.24).

Those operations have not been detailed on purpose; these surgeries correspond to about 5 % of indications and they are easier than you think.

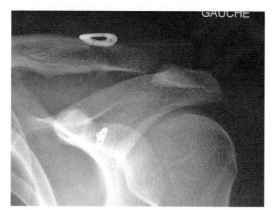

Fig. 6.17

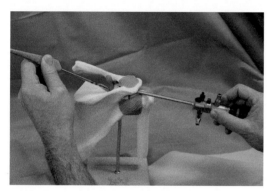

Fig. 6.18

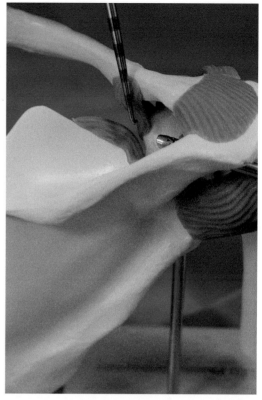

Fig. 6.19

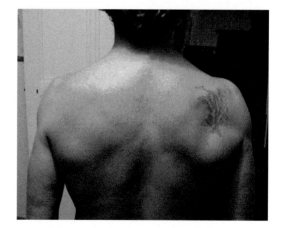

Fig. 6.20

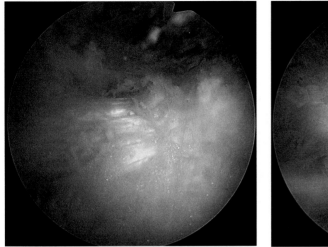

Fig. 6.21

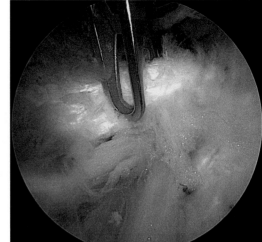

Fig. 6.23

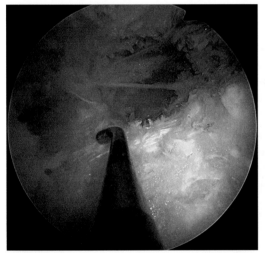

Fig. 6.22

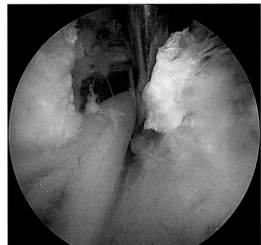

Fig. 6.24

How to Evolve Your Techniques

7

7.1 Analyze Your Mistakes, Travel, and Create

The evolution of techniques is necessary, but you have to be sure it will be also good for the patient.

It is from our failures that we evolve. Sometimes we have some difficulty in understanding them, or even seeing them. Either the failure is manifest like a recurrent dislocation; in this case, it is impossible to hide it unless we accuse the patient. Sometimes it is more subtle; the failure is not manifest, but regarding a certain technique, we do not feel completely at ease when we see the patients again.

Reviewing a series for a congress or in the context of a round table or symposium helps you to objectify your results and ask questions, especially when you are confronted by your colleagues.

This confrontation is necessary; it is good for the ego, it keeps you humble, and ultimately, it's good for the patient.

I will illustrate the point with some examples.

The handballer

At the time in 1994, Bankart surgery was already under discussion due to its recurrences. As a young unsuspecting surgeon, I began this surgery with conservative indications; this is how I gained more confidence and became bolder. This recurrence in a handballer challenged my optimism. One case was enough for me to ask questions and read the literature with different eyes (Fig. 7.1).

The lumberjack

Here again was an instability of the shoulder that I operated under arthroscopy. At the time, we grasped the labrum with a strong clamp and screwed the implant into the glenoid through the tissue. We did not see it; we recuperated our thread and performed a suture.

On the first visit, all went well, and on the second visit, the patient complained of noise in his

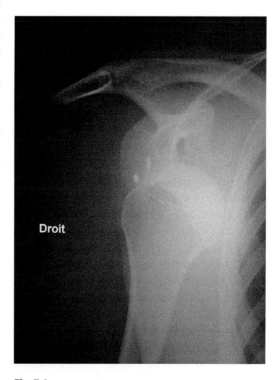

Fig. 7.1

© Springer International Publishing Switzerland 2015
O. Courage, *Shoulder Arthroscopy: How to Succeed!*, DOI 10.1007/978-3-319-23648-3_7

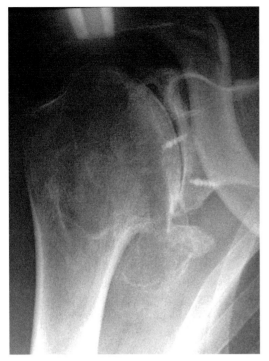

Fig. 7.2

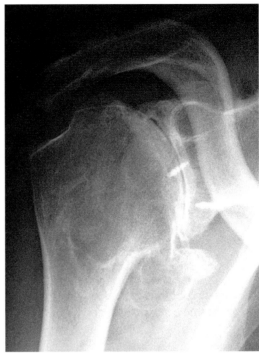

Fig. 7.3

shoulder. Always optimistic, I didn't panic. On the third visit, I did a scan on the patient; the implant was exceeding, so I removed it. Here are the results 10 years later (Figs. 7.2, 7.3, and 7.4).

Since then, I have never put an implant in without seeing it, and I immediately worry if a patient says to me that they have heard a noise in their shoulder.

The typical Normand

This case is more subtle. This is a typical patient in the region, and he even carries the name. I am close to him; we have common roots. In 2000, I operated a rotator cuff arthroscopy on him. The technique is simple and the results extraordinary. I was the "king of the world." The patient had an anterior elevation at 180°, no pain, and he was very satisfied. He was then integrated into the symposium on cuff repair. The MR arthrography showed a leaky cuff. This confrontation was salutary. The teamwork had revealed doubts about my technique, which I subsequently modified. Here is the famous slide of Mr Normand; he has never been re-operated on

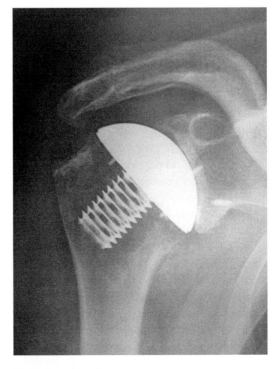

Fig. 7.4

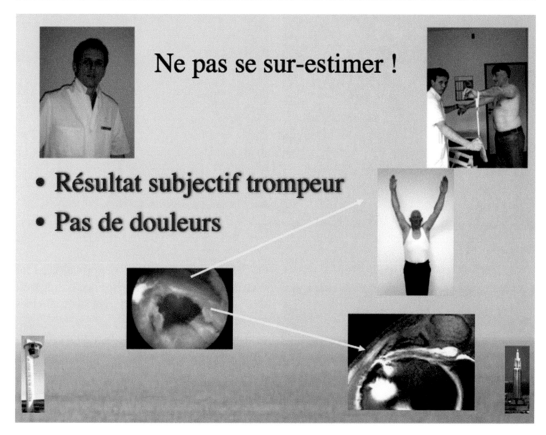

Fig. 7.5

and is still very happy with his shoulder even if he still has major doubts about my Jobe maneuver.

Here is the slide that has traveled extensively. If I had not done this symposium, I would have remained in my certainties (Fig. 7.5).

The friend's mother

Everything is good, the rotator cuff repair is well done, but I'll put an extra implant in to be safer because it's the mother of a friend.

Here is the result: now I never put an implant in if the view is insufficient and I check the incidence before proceeding.

We see in passing the importance of front and profile inspection radiologies (Figs. 7.6, 7.7, and 7.8).

The work accident

The patient worked as a warehouseman at the port, and on attempting to break a fall, he suffered

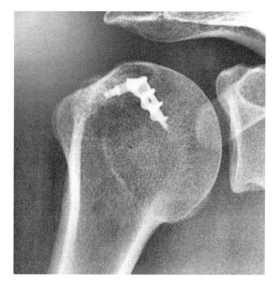

Fig. 7.6

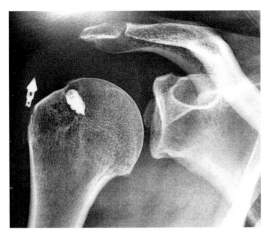

Fig. 7.7

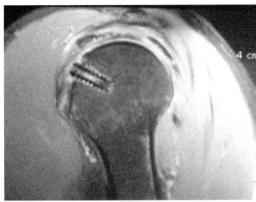

Fig. 7.9

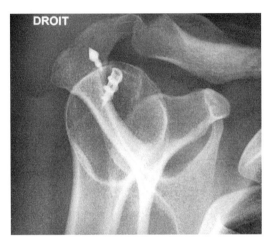

Fig. 7.8

a SLAP II biceps avulsion. I repaired the lesion arthroscopically; more than 6 months later, he still had pain, and he could not return to work. I took him in again for a tenodesis. At that time we did it intra-articularly above the groove, the biceps being fixed in a blind tunnel by an interference screw (Fig. 7.9).

On this implant lysis at more than 6 months, the patient was still in pain and still off work.

The case ended in a complaint….

I remained marked by this case; I am wary of SLAP, and since then, I do tenodeses under the groove.

You must know how to exploit failures to bounce back. You must not hide them and you must talk about them with colleagues. For me,

the SFA has always been a very good place for exchange. And as a "good Normand" I distrust these surgeons who are very sure of themselves and never have any problem.

Another way of evolving is to move around the obstacles.

This story is a bit long, but in hindsight, it makes me smile.

At the time, there was only one technique for cuffs under arthroscopy. We had to pass the wire with a well-known hook wheel. The industrials lent it to me, and I tried to repair the cuffs as best as I could, as had my predecessors.

But 1 day, they didn't want to lend it to me anymore. The clinic refused to buy it for me; I was not in favor with the "OR nurse chief".... There was no question for me give up these techniques, as I was sure that this was the future….

What do you do when you're confronted with a brick wall! The brain goes round and round to find a solution. This came to me at a moment when I was starting to despair. Adoring teaching, I used to enjoy listening to the SFA basic course the morning preceding the conference. It was when listening to Philippe Beaufils talk about meniscal sutures that the idea came to me.

The cuff is ultimately like a large meniscus. All you need to do is use a larger needle (Fig. 7.10).

From the next Monday, the anesthesiologist showed me a splendid spinal anesthesia needle. By bending it and passing it by all possible means, I could continue my rotator cuff repairs (Figs. 7.11, 7.12, and 7.13).

Fig. 7.10

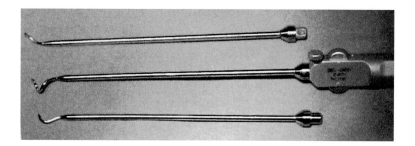

Fig. 7.11

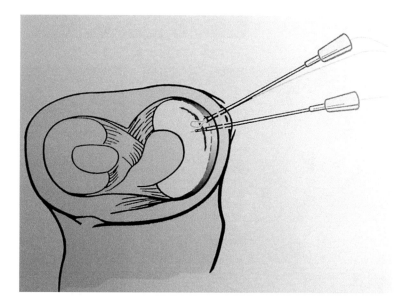

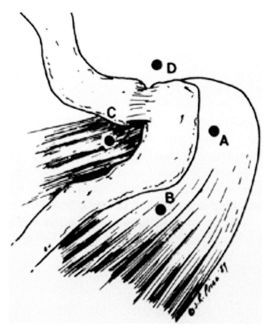

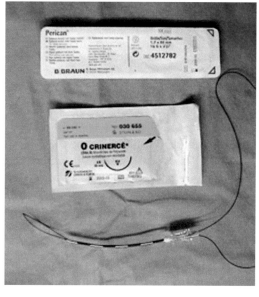

Fig. 7.13

Fig. 7.12

Fig. 7.14

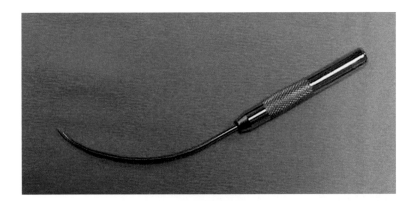

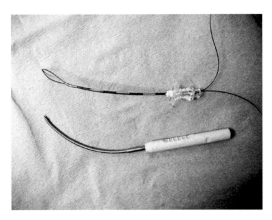

Fig. 7.15

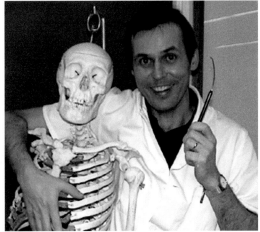

Fig. 7.16

I recovered good mood. But being a bit soft, the needle would bow from time to time, rendering the maneuver acrobatic.

I asked a company that was a competitor of the previous one to manufacture a solid needle with a handle. At that time, I never had the feeling of having invented anything. The prototype has evolved little (Figs. 7.14 and 7.15).

Then, when doing my first conference presentation, I took some punches that were well deserved. You don't change an "official" technique like that. You can't pass the tendon in this direction and above all there will be damage to the suprascapular nerve….

This nerve had hardly worried me at all. I could have ignored these criticisms, but I preferred to go further. I returned to the anatomy lab to "strengthen" my publication.

There was no danger as long as you were far enough back and at a distance from the dihedral angle. I admit that I should have started by this study (Figs. 7.16 and 7.17).

Now the Banana Lasso® is used worldwide. Here is Professor Yong Girl Rhee of South Korea who I met at the EITS of Taiwan! (Fig. 7.18)

I did not do things in the right order, but I cannot thank this block supervisor enough for being "blocked."

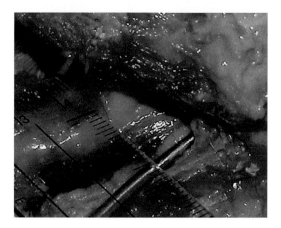

Fig. 7.17

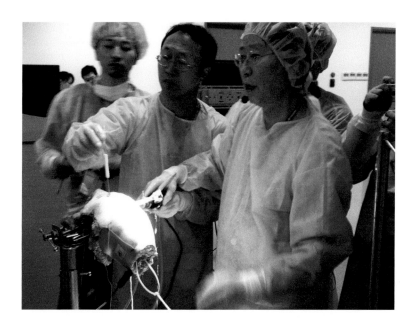

Fig. 7.18

Conclusion

Finally to finish this book, I think the best way to evolve is through human encounters that enrich us, provided you are open to them.

It would take pages to mention everyone; by prudence, I will not mention anyone, but all are acknowledged.

Firstly, I don't forget the solid surgical training with a boss (who asked me to do his shoulder) and his right arm, the king of arthroscopy in Caen. The atmosphere was familial and I even had the feeling of being treated like a son.

At the SFA, I always felt the support of a Parisian professor well before he became the president.

I attended my first symposium on rotator cuffs with the feeling of having entered a slightly more restricted circle. Neither of the two directors has ever looked down on me, even though I was from Le Havre!

During this symposium, I made the acquaintance of young people who have remained my friends ever since: speaker for my first morning conference on shoulder instability, my colleague who was so enthusiastic that we worked until 3 am to be fully prepared for the next day, and then the management of the symposium on the Bankart where I was able to work with a co-director who is a great man who has had the wisdom to remain simple.

Doing "science" in these conditions is extraordinary.

By listening to others, we sometimes modify our techniques.

Travel is always a source of enrichment. Like music (for surgeons who play the guitar), we are influenced. You should know to travel; techniques are learned in OR and not only by watching a video. You should know how to look at everything, sympathize with the teams, and also ask nurses for a reference for a wire that you have found to be very good that day. You must take photos and remember them in your old age; we always return from these trips starry-eyed.

© Springer International Publishing Switzerland 2015
O. Courage, *Shoulder Arthroscopy: How to Succeed!*, DOI 10.1007/978-3-319-23648-3

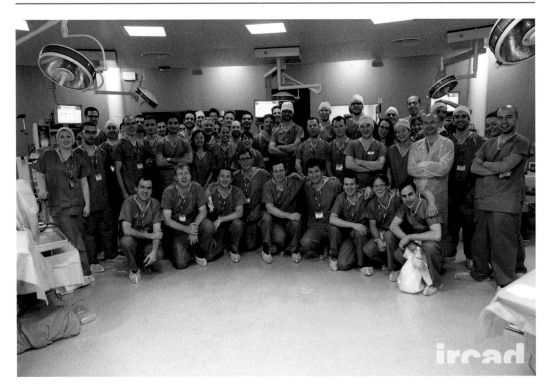

Fig. 1

Working with companies is not sufficiently valued. Yet their research facilities and training are often extraordinary. Without them, it would not be possible to evolve the techniques. They set up training for surgeons, and learning in these conditions and then becoming an instructor helps you to evolve in the right direction.

Besides, the surgeries that we perform directly (sometimes in acrobatic conditions) always leave us with good memories and allow us to glean other tricks.

I remember the Arthro live in Paris chaired by Philippe Hardy more than 10 years ago. Just before me, Steve Burkhart made a wonderful demo.

It was my turn… As you see in the picture he decided to stay in the OR. It's difficult to explain, I was under pressure with my nurse but rapidly, I felt something positive.

Steve was with me! At the end we talk together about techniques, he told me: "It's a nice idea to push sutures with the Banana lasso, then it's easy to retrieve them".

Even if you are a great surgeon as he is, if you have respect to the others you can learn small details from them.

Fig. 2

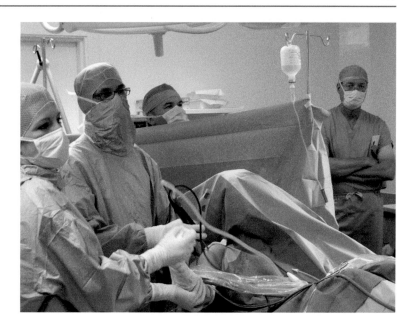

Visitors also offer us much because exchange between colleagues is interesting as well. I have counted 190 on the guest book! We thank them for making the trip to Normandy.

The training of young resident also and brings a great deal of satisfaction. We put our ideas in order so we can properly teach them. I think of all those who have come to train; I know they think of me during certain procedures in which I showed them "the trick."

Now some of them teach me new techniques.

For this, we need a good team. I thank my faithful nurses the "Couragettes" and particularly Safia who is the librarian of this book.

To conclude, I thank my wife Pascaline (her, I will mention), who has always left me free and understood this passion that is sometimes a bit too invasive. I would also like to

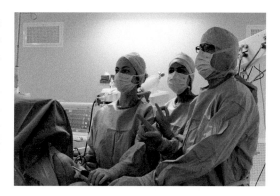

Fig. 3

kiss my three daughters; they have also been involved in this, and now they show me the example.

So that's it!